REDBOOK's

500 Sex Tips

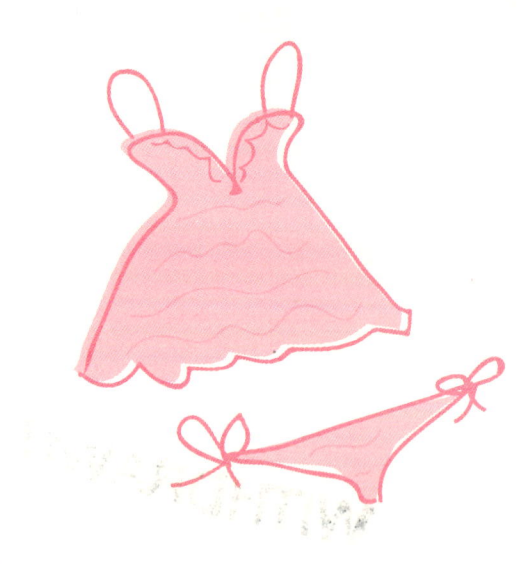

REDBOOK's

500 Sex Tips

How to Make Sex More Exciting, Satisfying & Fun

Judy Dutton

HEARST BOOKS
A division of Sterling Publishing Co., Inc.

New York / London
www.sterlingpublishing.com

Copyright © 2008 by Hearst Communications, Inc.

All rights reserved.

Library of Congress Cataloging-in-Publication Data
Dutton, Judy.
 Redbook's 500 sex tips : how to make sex more exciting,
satisfying & fun / Judy Dutton.
    p. cm.
 ISBN-13: 978-1-58816-662-3
 ISBN-10: 1-58816-662-7
 1. Sex instruction. 2. Sex. 3. Erotica. I. Redbook. II. Title.
 III. Title: 500 sex tips. IV. Title: Redbook's five hundred sex tips.
 HQ31.D94 2008
 613.9'6--dc22

                                                            2007029703

10 9 8 7 6 5 4 3 2 1

Published by Hearst Books
A Division of Sterling Publishing Co., Inc.
387 Park Avenue South, New York, NY 10016

Redbook and Hearst Books are trademarks
of Hearst Communications, Inc.

www.redbookmag.com

For information about custom editions, special sales, premium
and corporate purchases, please contact Sterling Special Sales
Department at 800-805-5489 or specialsales@sterlingpub.com.

Distributed in Canada by Sterling Publishing
c/o Canadian Manda Group, 165 Dufferin Street
Toronto, Ontario, Canada M6K 3H6

Distributed in Australia by Capricorn Link (Australia) Pty. Ltd.
P.O. Box 704, Windsor, NSW 2756 Australia

Manufactured in China

Sterling ISBN 13: 978-1-58816-662-3
          ISBN 10: 1-58816-662-7

BOOK DESIGN BY ALEXANDRA MALDONADO

CONTENTS

Introduction
Sex: Can it really be *that* good? • 7

CHAPTER 1
10 things you've been taught about sex that aren't true (phew!) • 9

CHAPTER 2
Get in a sexy state of mind • 19

CHAPTER 3
How to get *him* thinking about sex, too • 31

CHAPTER 4
Your sexy decorating to-do list • 39

CHAPTER 5
Dress for sex-cess • 43

CHAPTER 6
Get your sexercise! • 53

CHAPTER 7
Eat your way to better sex • 59

CHAPTER 8
Got a hot date? • 67

CHAPTER 9
Ladies, make your move! • 83

CHAPTER 10
12 totally new kisses to try on your guy • 93

CHAPTER 11
More foreplay, please! • 101

CHAPTER 12
Your head-to-toe guide to erogenous zones • 107

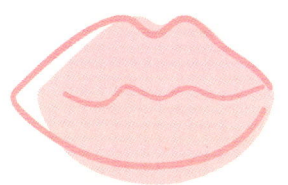
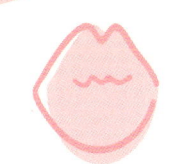

CHAPTER 13
Give him a hand! • 117

CHAPTER 14
How *he* can give *you* a hand • 127

CHAPTER 15
Blow him away! • 135

CHAPTER 16
The lowdown on going down • 143

CHAPTER 17
Assume the position! 22 to try • 151

CHAPTER 18
O my! Everything you need to know about orgasms • 161

CHAPTER 19
23 *very* sexy surprises • 175

CHAPTER 20
Sex toys: What's the buzz? • 185

CHAPTER 21
You wanna have sex *where*?! • 191

CHAPTER 22
The shy girl's guide to speaking up in bed • 201

CHAPTER 23
Fantasies: His, yours, and how to make them come true (if you want to) • 207

CHAPTER 24
Hey, what about romance? • 221

CHAPTER 25
Is your love life MIA? • 231

CHAPTER 26
Oops! 7 things you should never, ever try in bed • 249

Sources • 253
Index • 255

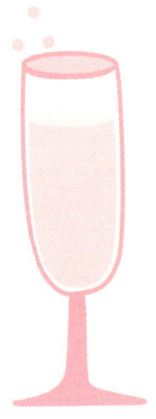

INTRODUCTION

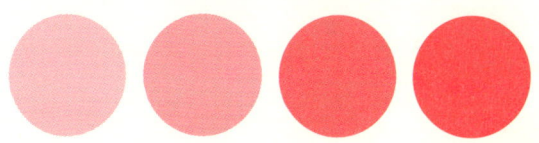

Sex: Can it really be *that* good?

Sex. No matter how many times you've had it, or which positions, techniques, toys, or crazy caped costumes you've tried, you can't help wondering: Is there more? Could it be even better? Well, we here at REDBOOK just couldn't help but weigh in: Yes. Or, more like *yes, yes, yes!* At least, that's our take after poring over millions of letters and e-mails from our readers through the years. In addition to being privy to the details of sexploits that normally wouldn't be discussed outside of the powder room, we also found women had questions. Like: *How can I have an orgasm during intercourse? What can I do if my husband wants sex every day, but I'm more of a once-a-week gal? Does horny goat weed really make you horny? And how can I keep the fireworks July 4th-worthy in spite of my kids/crazy schedule/the fact that we're doing it again, for the gazillionth time?*

Consider this book your guide to all of the above, and then some. Here, in one handy manual, we've gathered 500 of our top tips on how to make sex more satisfying, sensual, orgasmic, imaginative, and amazing than ever. Packed in these pages, you'll find wise advice from a range of sources—studies conducted by the nation's lead researchers, eye-opening REDBOOK polls, and plenty of illuminating insights straight from the mouths of men and women just like you—and chances are, once you've road-tested a few of these tricks, you'll see results, fast. Because let's face it, your love life is important. And it can be hard to keep things hopping. And yet, while most of us will happily consult a recipe before making polenta, or page through a manual to fix a glitch on our laptop, when it comes to sex, many of us just throw up our hands, turn off the lights, and hope for the best. If that sounds silly to you (and it should!), consider keeping this book within reach on your nightstand for your every nooky-related need, question, or concern . . . or just in case you and your guy are drawing a blank on what you could be doing with, to, or on top of each other tonight. We've got plenty of ideas.

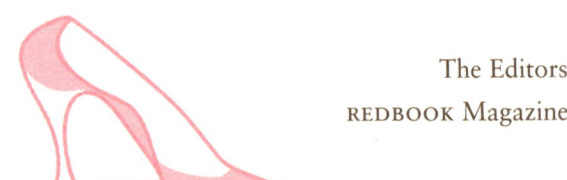

The Editors
REDBOOK Magazine

CHAPTER

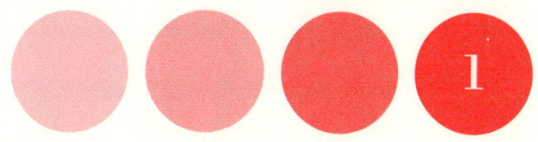

10 things you've been taught about sex that aren't true (phew!)

It's easy to think everyone's having hotter, wilder, crazier in-bed adventures than little old you. Between magazine cover lines like "Hour-long Orgasms!" and that single friend who spills *waaay* too much info about her one-night stands, any sane woman might wonder if she's the one dud in an undulating, ecstatic universe around her. But here's the thing: If you could take a peek inside couple's bedrooms right when they're going at it, you might be surprised to see how, well, normal it seems. There are sweet moments, steamy moments, awkward moments, stony silences, tentative hugs, so-so orgasms, no orgasms, inane giggles, pointless conversations about nothing in particular . . . such is the stuff that makes up this intimate slice of our lives. And believe it or not, it's true for all of us.

In other words, you can quit worrying: Whatever you're doing or feeling between the sheets, chances are you've got plenty of company. So let's set the record straight: Here are the top ten things women assume are true about sex that just don't click with what living, breathing couples are actually experiencing. Once it hits you how laughable these lovemaking myths truly are, it'll be easy to heckle them out of your life and start paying attention to what really matters: what you want. And once you get in touch with what pushes your buttons, you'll have the power to make your love life exactly what you want it to be—hot, wild, crazy, the works.

1

False fact: **Sex should be an earth-moving, angels-singing experience.**

Reality check: **Sometimes, sex is just sex.**

So you shot for an Oscar-worthy performance, but it ended up more like straight-to-video. Maybe one of you didn't cross the finish line, or got a foot cramp, or had *Did I take out the recycling?* spinning through your head nonstop. Hey, it happens. The strongest couples take these off-nights in stride—and definitely don't wait until the planets are perfectly aligned to try again (because honestly, how often do planets do that?). As a consolation prize, accept that even mediocre sex has its benefits. Maybe it resulted in a good laugh-and-cuddle afterward, or enabled you to burn off some energy and get a good night's sleep. That's worth something, don't you think?

2

False fact: **Sure sex is fun, but it's kind of a waste of time.**

Reality check: **Sex is good for you—really!**

Similar to flossing and seeing a shrink, shagging has been scientifically proven to enhance your physical and mental health.

So the next time you're thinking, *Don't we have more productive things to do than roll around?* keep these surprising perks in mind:

- Fewer sniffles. Duos who do the deed one to two times a week have 30 percent more flu-fighting antibodies than couples who copulate less than once a week, according to a study from Wilkes University in Wilkes-Barre, Pennsylvania.

- A slimmer waistline. Having an orgasm triggers the production of phenetylamine, a natural amphetamine that acts as an appetite suppressant.

- A healthier heart. Regular rolls in the hay improve your heart-rate fluctuation, an indicator of cardiovascular health.

- A youthful appearance. According to one study, women who get frisky three times a week look 7 to 12 years younger than their actual age.

- Improved fertility. Making whoopee at least once a week leads to higher rates of healthy ovulation.

- Less pain. Cramps and headaches will vanish, since the endorphins and oxytocin released during a tumble can increase your pain tolerance by as much as 70 percent.

- Dale Carnegie–level people skills. Physical intimacy hones your powers to tune into people's feelings and express your own—and not just with the guy in your bed but with everybody from your boss to your kids.

- Sunny disposition. The flood of hormones that accompanies orgasm helps reduce stress and improves your outlook. And the more often you hit a high note, the happier you'll be!

3

False fact: **Sex will happen when the mood strikes.**

Reality check: **Sometimes, you have to *make* the mood strike.**

Sure, it's nice when two people are inexorably drawn to each other and spontaneously combust like some madcap science experiment. But if you always hold out for that gotta-have-you-now feeling to hit *before* you grab each other, you may be waiting a very, very long time. Instead, try to jump-start your jonesing (we'll give you plenty of ideas on how to do that later), and occasionally, if he's hankering, consider giving it a go even when you aren't feeling inspired. Your mind may not be into it, but your body can be much easier to convince: A few knee-weakening kisses and caresses later, you could be raring to go.

4

False fact: **Men should make the first move.**

Reality check: **Why wait when you can pounce on him?**

Even after the sexual revolution, when word finally got out that women actually enjoy sex (duh!), men are still generally expected to be the ones to do the seducing while we ladies demurely sit by and wait for the invitations to roll in. But what if you want sex, like, *right now* while he's blissfully chatting about his workday? Step up to the plate and make a pass, and he'll be thrilled, *thrilled*, to see you lust for him the way he lusts for you. Meanwhile, you'll discover the joys of going for what you want, when you want it, and getting it. Talk about a power trip!

False fact: **You're too busy to have sex.**

Reality check: **If you care about your relationship, you'll find the time.**

Ask anyone how important it is to have a healthy, loving relationship, and most will say it's one of their top priorities. Look at how these very same people live their lives, though, and you'll see that intimacy often falls dead *last* on their to-do list. Sure, life is hectic. But don't be fooled, you make choices about how you spend your time. So if you find yourself saying, "I'll have sex after I get past this work deadline/help Junior finish his science project/organize the linen closet," try seeing it for what it is: "I'm *choosing* to put my career/kids/bath towels above a healthy, loving relationship." If you don't like how that sounds, then maybe it's time to reassess your schedule and see what can go so you can make room for what really matters in life: each other.

Girl talk tip-off

"I reminisce about the last time my husband and I had great sex—his touch, his breath on my skin, his sweet murmurings in my ear. By focusing on my sexiest memories, I'll bring myself to a fired-up state that often leads us into bed."

—Sasha, 36

Girl talk tip-off

"My husband is always the one to tug me toward the bedroom, and I've come to rely on his actions to get my motor running. But one evening, after putting the baby to bed, I walked up to my husband, grabbed his collar with both hands and pulled him in for the kiss of a lifetime—including full-body press and roving hands. He was so turned on by my assertiveness, the sex was amazing. That role swap was like an erotic awakening for both of us."

—Jenny, 35

6

False fact: **Great sex lasts for hours.**

Reality check: **Great sex can be as short—or as long—as you want.**

Sure, it'd be great if you had tons of time carved out to light a shrine's worth of candles and make love 'til the cows come home. But let's get real: For most of us, that opportunity comes around, oh, almost never. That's why for busy couples today, the smart move is to bust out of the two-hours-on-Saturday-night mindset and grab opportunities whenever you can find them. If that ends up being a four-minute window between when he sets foot in the door and the start of *Grey's Anatomy*, so be it. Get moving!

7

False fact: **Sex = intercourse.**

Reality check: **Sex = whatever floats your boat.**

The conventional wisdom is that once you hit a home run, you can't be satisfied just hanging out on bases one through three. But these days, smart couples realize that sex encompasses not only intercourse, but any kind of activity that turns you on. This insight is especially important for women, many of whom don't regularly reach orgasm via the old bump 'n' grind. So if you prefer to stick with oral maneuvers or make out like teenagers all night, that's fine and dandy, and don't let anyone tell you otherwise.

SURPRISING SEX FACT!

Working-age Americans have gained, rather than lost, free time since 1965—between four and eight hours a week, according to a study by the Federal Reserve Bank of Boston. Maybe you and your guy should consider spending one of those hours in bed (and not sleeping, either).

False fact: At this point, you've got his turn-ons down pat.

Reality check: His (and your) turn-ons are a moving target.

Maybe today you're both into woman-on-top positions and dirty talk. Tomorrow it could be sex toys and him in a Santa suit. Our point is, people's desires evolve over the years, and the only way to continue hitting the bull's-eye is to keep asking and exploring. Even if most of your experiments fizzle, you'll have fun trying. And who knows? One or two may be such successes that you'll shout "Eureka!" and then some. Now, who said sex (or your sweetie) isn't full of surprises?

False fact: Giving directions in bed will undermine his male ego.

Reality check: Giving directions will boost his ego by letting him know he's on track.

It may be a running joke that men refuse to ask for directions while driving, but when it comes to *your* terrain, most will fully admit they're lost—which is why a few pointers like "slower," "faster," "a little to the right/left" followed by an "ooh, yeah, don't stop!" are always appreciated. That way, you're happy, and that means he's happy, and maybe next time, he'll head down these avenues on his own. (Note: Don't fake it! That's like putting up a sign saying "Orgasm: this way!" down a dead-end path.)

> ### Girl talk tip-off
>
> "Fast sex can be amazing. Maybe we have 10 minutes before the kids come home, or five minutes in the kitchen before guests arrive—suddenly we're discovering how to have sex on the big chopping-block island."
>
> —Elizabeth, 36

10

False fact: **The fireworks fade over time.**

Reality check: **Sex doesn't get dull until the day you stop trying.**

We won't lie to you, the fireworks do fade *a little*. And good thing, too. If they didn't, you'd never make it out of bed long enough to pay your bills, feed your pets/kids, or show up to work on time because you'd be too busy burrowing into each other as if the meaning of life were buried somewhere between you. Instead, thank goodness, you can relax a little once the initial red-hot attraction cools a bit. But relax *too* much, and is it any head-scratcher why you're no longer burning up the bedsheets? Think back to when you two first started dating. We'll bet you spent eons getting dolled up before meeting him, giggled at his jokes (even the bad ones), and went all out to weave your spell and ensure the sex you'd soon be having would knock his boxer shorts off. Bring back just one-tenth of the effort you expended during your early days, and we think you'll be pleasantly surprised to see sparks fly. No, you may no longer be getting off on that amazing new-guy smell or those thrilling new-guy sound effects, but at this point you have something much, much more valuable: a man you trust. That means you can take him anywhere. And with sex, there are so many places to go.

SURPRISING SEX FACT!

Studies estimate that the first intense phase of love lasts one to three years on average. After that, the hormonal high that kept you hornier than a brass band dies down somewhat. Consider this nature's way of conserving some energy for other pursuits, like eating, sleeping, and raising the kids that may have come about as a result of all your mischief.

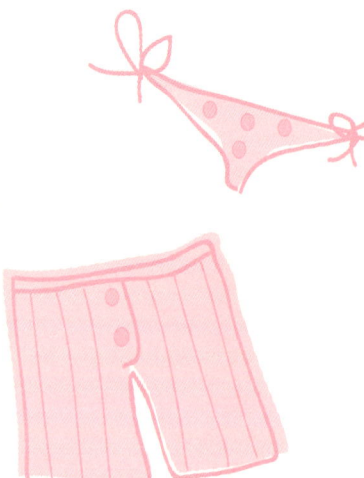

CHAPTER

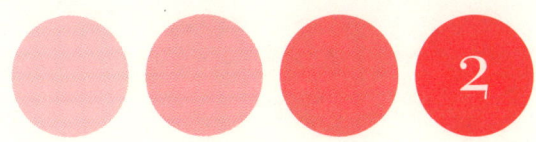

Get in a sexy state of mind

So what's the first step to having an incredible sex life? Well, the answer's so simple we almost feel silly saying it: You've gotta think about sex—and not just when you're a few slipper shuffles away from bed, either. Make an effort to see the sensual silver lining in every occasion, no matter how small, and it's bound to get those gears turning. Let this chapter clue you in to all the ways you can walk, talk, and think in a slightly more risqué way. Adopt just a few of these habits, and the world may suddenly seem a lot more interesting.

One woman's sex secret—revealed

"Nothing makes me feel sexier than indulging myself. Whether it's having my legs waxed on my lunch hour or buying a tiny bag of very expensive chocolates to eat on the train home, an indulgence makes me feel pampered, sexy. When I see my husband, I want to ravish him."

—Jana, 29

11 Give yourself a secret sexy alias

Pick a new name for yourself, and make it a good one (meaning it should sound like it belongs in a James Bond flick—Bambi or Natasha, for instance). This, ladies, is your alter ego. She's here to make it easy for you to mentally switch gears from everyday you to Seductress Extraordinaire. Just ask yourself, "How would Bambi handle this situation?" and you may be surprised what this dark angel on your shoulder tempts you to do.

12 Strut your stuff

If you're galumphing through the grocery store aisles, no wonder you're not feeling like much of a minx. Add some boom-chick-a to your walk, though, and your mind is sure to follow. Here's how: Tuck your pelvis under your torso so your lower body forms a concave arc, then throw back your shoulders and stick out your chest. Put one foot right in front of the other and it'll force your hips to naturally shaboom-shaboom from side to side. Add a runway model pout, and voilà, the world is your catwalk.

13   Do something decadent

Every few weeks, take 10 bucks of "play money" and throw it at something frivolous: Pamper yourself with a pedicure. Buy a bouquet of fresh flowers. Nibble on a small can of caviar or a tiny box of truffles. Why? Because you're worth it, that's why! And by regularly affirming your VIP status, you may start spoiling yourself in, ahem, other ways.

14   Learn to love a compliment

When someone says, "That dress looks amazing on you," do you blush and downplay the remark with a self-deprecating "Oh, this old thing? I've had it for years . . . "? Hel-*lo*, someone just paid you a compliment! Accept it. Believe it. Say "Thank you! You just made my day!" Then *let* it make your day.

SURPRISING SEX FACT!

Exercise pumps up your ego: According to one study, 60 percent of women who work out two to three days a week—and 88 percent of those who do so four to five days a week—consider themselves more attractive than the average gal.

One woman's sex secret—revealed

"To boost my libido, I indulge in erotic thinking: I might see a pile of peaches in the supermarket and let my mind drift to imagine them as glorious bottoms, male and female. When I think about my husband, I sometimes picture parts of him, like his forearm or chest hair; I visualize that part until I feel aroused. Even the most mundane things can have an erotic appeal. Running my hand along a curved wooden banister can be a sensual experience."

—Nicola, 28

15 Hit the gym

Of course, staying fit will make you feel like a fox. But believe it or not, you don't have to wait until you've dropped a size to feel sexy; the mental benefits can kick in after merely one or two workouts. That's because making an effort to improve or to care for your bod, no matter how small, can instantly improve your confidence levels *and* your willingness to flaunt the fruits of your labors.

16 Stop censoring your sexy thoughts

Ever been standing in line, stuck in traffic, or otherwise biding your time and felt your mind wander in some dirty direction? Whether you're mulling over the great sex you had that morning or some kinky fantasy you've yet to try, go ahead and dwell on it rather than shoving it aside as silly daydreaming. Your imagination is the fuel that powers real-life passion, so it's in your best interest to keep that mental motor running.

17 Start a sex diary

Alas, some of our most titillating thoughts flash through our minds so fast they're quickly forgotten. The solution? Keep a notebook handy to jot them down as they fly by. Entries can be as short as *I can't wait for my guy to get home from work today so I can_____* [fill in the blank], or maybe you've got a Harlequin novel's worth of smoldering storylines just waiting to spill from your subconscious. Either way, by putting them to paper, you prevent them from fading away any time soon.

18 Take catcalls in stride

Like it or not, whistling construction workers are a fact of life, which means you have two choices: (a) give them mean looks and let them ruin your day, or (b) accept that they're merely appreciating your damn fine ass. Now, which sounds more fun?

SURPRISING SEX FACT!

Think women take a while to get aroused? Not according to a study by Stanford University, which found that female subjects took only two minutes to get sexually charged.

19   Pick your own personal theme song

Choose one that makes you feel soulful, sensual, unstoppable. (Some suggestions: the Rolling Stones' "Start Me Up" or Aretha Franklin's "You Make Me Feel Like a Natural Woman.") Then, any time you need a shot of va-va-voom, blast it—in your car, your home, your head—for an instant pick-me-up.

20   Learn to look at yourself through rose-tinted goggles

We know, it's hard to feel like hot stuff when you're obsessed with your thunder thighs or that wrinkle under your armpit. But it's your mind, not your bod, that needs the overhaul here, and all that's required is a small shift in focus. Rather than obsessing about the body parts you hate, hone in on things you *love*, like your killer legs, eyes, or smile. That's easier said than done, we know, but keep practicing, and over time it'll become second nature and you'll actually begin to believe what you see.

Girl talk tip-off

"I consciously add some zing to all different little areas in my life. I do things like wear silky undies, buy myself an ice cream cone and eat it really suggestively, or take the most luxurious shower before work with all sorts of scrubs and creams. They keep that erotic energy in me at a constant hum."

—Amanda, 35

One woman's sex secret—revealed

"I indulge in frequent adulterous fantasies to keep my libido high. Driving in the car to work, riding in an elevator, waiting on line, or pumping my own gas, I weave little erotic stories around men I know or happen to see. A construction worker with bulging biceps becomes my secret lover. We're having sex standing up with my legs wrapped around his waist while he runs the jackhammer with one hand."

—Andrea, 41

21 Go ahead and notice guys

Ever heard a man say, "I'm married, not dead" when trying to explain how he can love his wife but his head still swivels every time some hottie breezes by? Well, he's got a point: Appreciating the eye candy around you can make you feel more alive. And if some man-hunk you're admiring inspires you to jump your own guy this evening, honestly, what's the harm?

22 Flirt up a storm with strangers

So the aforementioned man-hunk is eyeing you right back? Even if you're happily taken, that doesn't mean you can't bask in a little male attention. Go ahead and raise an eyebrow, or giggle with the waiter, or that traffic cop who pulled you over, or that cute guy who mistakenly picked up your Chinese take-out instead of his. It's fun, it's an ego boost, and it's good practice for how you should be treating your own sweetie. (After all, who said you should stop working your wiles once you know he's probably not going anywhere?)

23 Find your trigger fragrance

Scent and sexuality are closely linked, so go ahead and explore which aromas get a rise out of you. Don't limit yourself to candles and cologne—maybe you love the smell of sweat and gasoline on your guy's T-shirt, or freshly cut grass, or laundry hot out of the dryer. Breathe deep and you may be surprised where your mind wanders.

24 Take a time-out

Don't get us wrong, nothing beats being surrounded by the people you love. But sitting with your own thoughts for a spell—in a café flipping through a celebrity rag, seeing a movie your guy would watch only to humor you—will help you cut through the noise and needs of others and get you back in touch with your own mental patter. Refreshed and centered, you'll return to the swing of things all the more ready to reach out to others, including the guy giving you a welcome-home hug.

Girl talk tip-off

"No matter how busy I am, I schedule some time just for me. No husband, kids, friends, work—just me. I may send the kids to the park for two hours with my husband on Saturday morning so I can stay in bed and read a book, or hire a sitter and go to a foreign-language film. Occasional time-outs restore me. I feel sexy, like a woman who has an interesting life of her own. In my mind, I am coming to him as an intriguing stranger."

—Carolyn, 31

SURPRISING SEX FACT!

Strange, but true: The Smell & Taste Treatment and Research Foundation in Chicago found that the smell of Good & Plenty candy increases vaginal blood flow by 14 percent. For men, a combo of lavender and pumpkin pie increases penile blood flow by 40 percent.

25   Clock more time in your birthday suit

Why? Because if you're at all bashful about your body, stripping down more often will get you so used to baring all you'll eventually forget to feel self-conscious. So go ahead and fold the laundry, read a book, or pay your bills au naturel (or, if privacy is an issue, wear a bikini and/or keep a robe handy). By merely exposing yourself to exposure more often, you'll shoot your sexual self-confidence through the roof.

26   Master the art of foot self-massage

According to the ancient Chinese art of reflexology, your foot contains thousands of nerve endings that, if pressed the right way, can get your whole body humming from head to toe with renewed sexual energy. Sure, it would be nice if we all had our own personal foot masseuses at our beck and call, but until that happens, here's how you can do it yourself. Place your thumbs near the center of the sole of your foot, then slowly walk them

> ## >> Inside the male mind
>
> *"I think my wife is totally hot. She'll point out what she perceives as flaws, but I think she's nuts. Even if I'm not in the mood, I'll catch a glimpse of her taking off her bra, and bam! I'm in the mood. Which is great at night, but slightly problematic in the morning if she's trying to throw some clothes on to make her train."*
>
> —Dan, 31

up diagonally toward your big and pinkie toes. Then, use your thumbs to stroke the arch. Finish off by slightly rotating each toe between thumb and forefinger to put a spring in your step.

27   Slowly brush your hair

...as you daydream about him running his hands through your hair. It'll up the chances you'll be hankering to have it happen for real later.

28   Strategize your next seduction

Got time to kill before your guy arrives home? Make good use of it by imagining exactly how you're going to put the moves on him tonight. Visualize how it'll happen, frame by frame: He's chopping carrots, you slip behind him, languidly let your hands wander from his chest, down, down into the top of his pants . . . Now, replay this steamy scenario over and over. Once the opportunity arises to put your plan into action, you'll feel more fired up than a Bond girl on a mission.

29   Savor your senses

Breathe deeply of the flowers that others merely sniff. Close your eyes and really linger over every bite of that hot fudge sundae. Tune into the simple pleasures brimming in the world around you, and a more sensual mindset will soon become second nature, in bed and out.

Girl talk tip-off

"I didn't feel sexually desirable when my pregnancy began showing, but I didn't want to spend the next six months refusing my husband's advances. A book about goddesses inspired me: Many of the goddess figures were, frankly, fat, with big bellies. I bought a clay figure shaped like one of them and made an altar to her with candles, an incense holder, and flowers. To put myself in the mood for love, I lit candles and incense and spent a few minutes meditating before my goddess altar. I still use it sometimes."

—Amy, 31

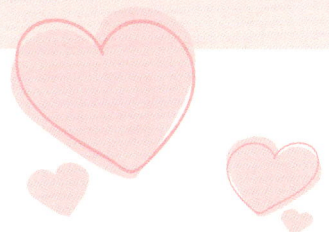

30 Try seeing yourself through your guy's eyes

Men, bless their simple, Homer Simpson–style hearts, are amazingly easy to please in pretty much all areas of life. Never is this truer than when he looks at you. So the next time your sexual self-confidence is sagging, consider what *he'd* be thinking if your bare bod were within his sights. Chances are, it would be something along the lines of *Wow, gorgeous*. Period. And honestly, if he's not nitpicking, why should you?

Girl talk tip-off

"The standard advice is: Flirt with your husband to keep the attraction alive. There's nothing wrong with that. But lighthearted flirting with a stranger, a coworker, or a male friend also gets the juices going. An exchange of smiles, compliments, and flirty gestures with an attractive man makes me feel desirable. I want to go home and make love to my husband after another man's eyes have lingered on my body."

—Tina, 34

CHAPTER

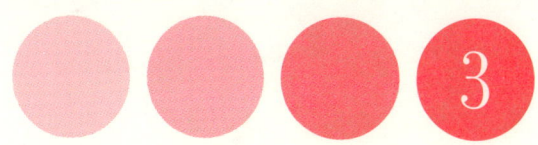

How to get *him* thinking about sex, too

We know what you're probably thinking right now: *A whole chapter devoted to getting my guy riled up? He's already riled up enough, thank you.* You have a point. Still, admit it: While we often take it for granted that guys go gaga at the slightest encouragement, there are days when even he can feel overworked, underappreciated, and could use a reminder that, hey, life isn't *that* bad, he's got a sexual dynamo sharing his toothpaste! We've come up with a slew of clever ways you can keep him in an I-want-her-now heat from morning 'til night. Because deep down, as much as we gripe about how guys are always all over us, honestly, where would our egos be without *them*?

31 Whisper "Buon giorno, amore mio" to him in the a.m.

"Good morning" never sounded so suggestive.

32 Slay him with a stretch

You know, that one where you casually lift your arms up straight above your head and hold while arching your back a bit, thus lifting your boobs and exposing a hint of midriff. So sexy.

33 Share a sexy dream

Mention, casually, while he's brushing his teeth or you're pouring your coffee, "You know, I had a really interesting dream last night." Then describe a favorite fantasy of yours. Spare no detail: where you were, how he touched you, the works. He'll hold that image in his head for a *long* time.

34 After your shower, flash him fast...

Do it so quickly he'll think it was all in his (dirty) mind.

35 ... Or flash him slow

Make your intentions all too apparent by flinging your towel wide open. Ask him to picture you—just like this—all day long. This catch-him-off-guard come-on will make him wish he could call in sick and feast his eyes on you all day.

Girl talk tip-off

"I do things in the morning that get him lusting after me. A stretch while I'm getting dressed, where I raise my arms and stick my chest out in front of him, does wonders. I give him an eyeful that he reruns in his mind all day. Sex is inevitable that evening."

—Diana, 34

SURPRISING SEX FACT!

What's the sexiest part of a woman's body? According to a REDBOOK survey, 35 percent of men voted for breasts, with an equal number rallying for your rear end; 17 percent love a woman's mouth, while 13 percent admire your nether regions the most.

36 Help him get dressed

Mention his boxers look a little twisted—then do a hands-on readjustment. Having his own personal undies stylist is guaranteed to get a rise out of him, so to speak.

37 Treat him to a reverse striptease

Sure, men are used to sneaking a peek when you take it all off. Getting garbed up, though, can make him equally speechless. First up: your panties. Turn your back to him, step into a pair, then do that little butt shimmy—where you move your legs like you're climbing a ladder—as you pull them up. Next, the bra: Slip your arms into the straps and arch your back as you reach behind and do the clasp; then use your hands to maneuver your breasts in the cups, fondling them way longer than necessary. Putting on hose? Perch one leg on a chair, slip the stockings over your foot and very slowly ease them up, making sure to stroke and caress your gams as you go. Do it all without glancing his way. He'll get a voyeuristic kick if you pretend you don't notice him ogling, even though you know better.

SURPRISING SEX FACT!

What's the sexiest part of a man's body? According to a poll by REDBOOK, 42 percent of women say his chest. His kissable lips and squeezable behind tie for second at 24 percent, while a no-nonsense 10 percent say his package takes the cake.

38   Admire your assets

It's unanimous: Men hate it when women ask, "Does this outfit make me look fat?" It's also unanimous that men *love* when women ask, "Doesn't this skirt make my butt look incredible?" or "Does this top give me cleavage that just won't quit?" Not only do these comments exude sexy self-confidence, you're calling attention to something well worth appreciating.

39   And while you're at it, check him out

When he's getting dressed, let him catch you giving him The Look—you know, that up-and-down stare that all but says you want to eat him for breakfast. Then say, "You look hot in that suit" or just shake your head, saying "Mm-mm." It'll make his day, and may fuel some studly behavior later.

40   Spritz your perfume on something he takes to work . . .

That way, even when you're miles apart, you can remind him of what it's like to be close to you . . . and get him wishing he could be even closer.

41 . . . Or give him a racy photo to go

Take a picture of yourself, wrapped in nothing but a white sheet. On the back, write "A little reminder of what's waiting for you when you get home," then slip it into his suitcase or coat pocket before he leaves.

42 Give him a delicious good-bye kiss . . .

He's off to work and has leaned in for the standard *sayonara* smooch. Surprise him by going beyond your usual peck on the lips and make this kiss count: Part your lips, close your eyes, and enjoy it. Accompanied with a sexy purr or playful "Seeya later, stallion," it will linger in his mind all day.

43 . . . And an equally enthusiastic "Welcome home, honey"

Throw your arms around him and lock lips as if he's been away not just for the day, but years. At war. Show him how thrilled you are he's back and you may have *quite* a reunion on your hands.

Moves men love

"When Cassie's in the mood for lovemaking or for reminding me how sexy she is, she makes sure I see her undress. After raising her skirt above her thighs, she removes her stockings, running her hands along her calves as she pulls them down. Then she slowly unbuttons her blouse, giving me sexy looks between each button. Finally, she undoes her bra and cups her breasts as the straps fall off her shoulders. It makes me nuts."

—John, 40

44 Move in slow motion

True temptresses take their sweet time doing everything—ambling across a room, sipping a glass of wine, pausing a beat to think, then respond, to a question. Try it around your guy to capture his attention, and keep it.

45 Talk dirty during daylight hours

Give even your most casual conversations an eyebrow-raising edge by tossing in a few titillating terms. Even if you're just talking about how "arousing" the warm breeze feels on your skin this evening or what a "turn-on" it is when he does the cooking, this sort of unexpected lusty lingo can instantly fuel the mood.

46 Invade his personal space

It's simple: Just have your conversation with him one foot closer than usual. Is he having trouble finishing his sentences? That's due to the sexual chemistry brewing between you.

47 Flirt with your eyes

It's easy: Tuck your chin down, then slowly let your peepers travel up to meet his so you're peering through your top lashes. This coquettish, come-hither glance is so bewitching he's bound to start salivating.

Girl talk tip-off

"One morning I woke up and told him about a sexy dream I had about us. This led to a heavy lovemaking session. He does not ever need to know that I made it all up!"

—Jen, 31

> ### Moves men love
>
> "One time when we were watching a video on the sofa, she laid her head on my lap, took my hand and slowly kissed each of my fingers, keeping her eyes locked on mine the whole time. There was no mistaking what was on her mind, so I paused the movie."
>
> —Mike, 37

48 Give him a surprise peek

During dinner, lean in to grab the salt and give him a peek at your cleavage. Hike up your skirt and scratch some make-believe itch on your thigh. If he assumes it was a lucky accident, why bother correcting him?

49 Say it softly

Whatever you have to get off your chest, sidle up and whisper it in his ear, even if it's merely to murmur, "Want more wine with dinner, baby?" That breathless baby-doll voice did wonders for Marilyn Monroe and can for you, too.

50 Sit on his lap

Perch your pretty little derriere on his thighs while he's reading the paper, watching *Monday Night Football*, or whenever he looks like he'd least appreciate a distraction. Align your backside just so and shift your weight every so often so you're comfortable . . . and he isn't.

51 Pose like a Parisian artist's muse

While watching TV, recline on the sofa on your side with your head propped up on one hand and one leg crossed at the knee in front of the other. This sultry move thrusts your chest out and accentuates your hips. And that means that no matter what's on TV, you're probably his entertainment for the evening.

52 Reach out and touch . . . yourself

It's body language 101: If you want your man to look at something, touch it. Caress your neck. Fiddle with an earring. Adjust your bra straps. Twist a strand of your hair between your fingers. And watch his eyes follow your every move.

53 Sneak a peek at his package

Let your gaze repeatedly wander down, down, down . . . When he catches on, make it clear that you like what you see with an I-can't-help-myself shrug and a smile. Reminding him that he's got it (and you want it) is the ultimate compliment.

54 Go ahead and get comfortable

Casually unclasp your bra and pull it out your sleeve, like Jennifer Beals did in *Flashdance*. Don't be surprised if his hands start wandering.

55 Wear full PJs to bed

Then strip in the middle of the night. Trust us, it'll make his morning.

CHAPTER 4

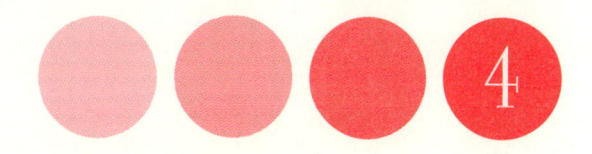

Your sexy decorating to-do list

Look around you. If you're at home, you'd probably admit that, barring a few annoyances like the stack of mail on the kitchen counter or the load of laundry that needs folding, you feel pretty comfortable in your surroundings. But do you feel sexy? Probably not. After all, your tastes may run more toward shabby chic or midcentury modern than Playboy mansion. Still, while a mirror on the bedroom ceiling or eyebrow-raising sculptures may be so not your style, we'd like to suggest some subtle modifications that'll add a little more ambience (and don't worry, we're talking really subtle—only you will notice the difference). A more sumptuous backdrop, after all, can help set the stage for some really hot sex, so try adding few of these elements to your bedroom, then watch the temperature rise.

SURPRISING SEX FACT!

85 percent of women admit they get a rise out of reading bodice rippers, according to one survey.

56 A dimmer switch

If your current lighting options during sex boil down to pitch black or a harsh 100-watt glare, a dimmer switch is probably the best five bucks you'll ever spend. Now you can adjust the brightness so you can have *some* eye candy, but not *so* much that you can count each other's pores. Huge, huge improvement.

57 Red light bulbs . . .

They'll bathe the room (not to mention your bod) in a gorgeous warm glow. Less messy than candles but just as seductive!

58 . . . Or a red scarf

Drape it over your bedside lamp and a rosy, bordelloesque ambience awaits.

59 A CD player on your nightstand

Having mood-setting music within arm's reach of the bed will definitely come in handy, so invest in a small CD player and you can pick what to listen to rather than be at the whim of what's on your alarm clock radio. Morning traffic reports? *So* not a turn-on.

60   A potted pink orchid on each side of the bed

There's a reason why Georgia O'Keeffe's myriad orchid canvases look so much like a certain part of the female anatomy: These are shockingly sexy flowers. Their mere presence should stir a little creative coupling.

61   A revved-up reading list

Sure, those bodice rippers stashed by the checkout aisle may look a little over-the-top, but take a peek at these guilty pleasures and you'll see why: They're perfect fodder for what you and your own Fabio could be doing once you can bring yourself to set them aside. (If you truly need something more literary, try Anaïs Nin's *Delta of Venus* or *The Story of O* by Pauline Réage.)

62   Bed sheets that beg you to stay in bed

Go for bust and buy the best: Egyptian cotton. The higher the thread count, the finer the weave—and the more amazing they'll feel to roll around in. As the saying goes, you spend one-third of your life in bed. Why not entice yourself to linger a little longer?

63   Colors that'll get you hot under the collar

Can the right hues heat things up? Absolutely. To create an undress-me ambience, make sure your bed sheets, curtains and walls are awash in warm colors like deep red or dark orange. Steer clear of cold colors such as white or mint green, which can put passion on ice.

64 — The power of feng shui in your corner

According to this ancient Eastern art, arranging furniture and objects a certain way can generate *chi*, or positive energy. To get those good vibes flowing, reposition your bed so your feet don't face the door. Then, locate your bedroom's "relationship" area (the far right corner as seen from the door or back wall), remove any clutter, and place a pair of red candles there, which should light up your love life in no time.

Plus: 4 things that'll sex up your bathroom

65 — A full-length mirror

Seeing yourself full-frontal every time you step out of the shower will keep other naked activities on your brain (ditto for him).

66 — A translucent shower curtain

That way, every time you suds up, you'll be giving your guy a tantalizingly blurry image of you.

67 — Big fluffy towels

A touch of luxury helps set an indulgent mood.

68 — A big, spalike candle on the tub

Even if you almost never light the thing, it's a subliminal reminder of another way to put your master bath to good use (wink, wink).

CHAPTER 5

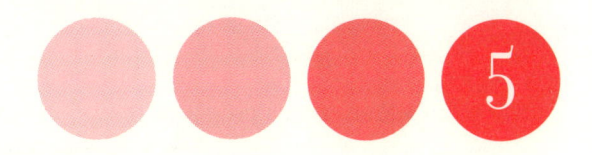

Dress for sex-cess

If sex is a gift everyone loves to get, then the clothes you wear are the pretty packaging. And no doubt about it, dressed just right, you can get a guy dying to unwrap the goods. Of course, we women know this instinctively, which is why we shop for hours, days, and weeks for the perfect outfit and lacy underthings that'll make us feel hot to trot. But while it's easy to assume you need a huge wardrobe allowance to look like a million bucks, we're here to tell you that sometimes, it's the *tiniest* tweaks to what you wear—and bare—that can transform you into a bombshell. Just mix and match a few of these tips, plus a few of the extra-foxy hair and makeup tricks we threw in for good measure, and you'll exude so much me-so-sexy magnetism that chances are those clothes won't stay on for long (nor will you want them to).

69 — Invest in some little black undies

You already know that a little black dress is a crucial component of any gal's wardrobe. Well, here's another essential: a barely-there lace bikini or thong in *noir*. Now you'll never be at a loss for what to wear *under* that little black dress, or be shy about showing it off.

70 — Put on clothes that say "pet me"

Silk, suede, cashmere, faux fur . . . unlike your usual cotton duds, these materials feel amazing against your skin and beg to be caressed. Talk about an easy way to get your guy's hands all over you.

71 — Wear jewelry where you normally wouldn't

A belly chain, a toe ring, an upper-arm cuff . . . once these shiny objects have captured his attention, use your creativity to keep it.

72 — Lay on the eyeliner

Slightly smudged black eyeliner = smoldering sexpot. Put it on. Look in the mirror. Feel like doing something very, very bad tonight? We thought so.

73 — Glam up your hands . . .

Manicures turn everyday mitts into instruments of mass seduction. Suddenly, every gesture you make seems mesmerizing; every object, person, or (ahem) body part you touch gets stroked in a more sensual way.

74 . . . Or get a set of ridiculously long press-on nails

Granted, they might be impractical to wear on a daily basis. But if you save them for the right occasion, wow do they make you look like a minx! Wear them on a weekend when you know manual labor isn't on your agenda and see what these talons tempt you to do.

75 Let your hair down

During dinner or whenever he least expects it, let your hair slip out of its updo to generate some major sex-kitten appeal.

76 Break your lingerie out of the boudoir

If you tend to think of lingerie as something you wear only while lounging in bed as your guy looks on, we can only ask: Why? That slinky camisole or see-through bra-and-panty can (and should!) be worn any old day you need a mental lift—just put them on under your regular clothes and no one will be the wiser. Simply knowing that your inner bombshell is lying one layer beneath your business suit can get you into a smokin' I-have-a-secret mindset, and think how pleasantly surprised *he'll* be when you start shedding your layers later that night.

77 Transport yourself to the tropics

Wear a sprig of freesia or jasmine in your hair to feel incredibly island-sexy all day. Smells yummy and looks even yummier.

dress for sex-cess

78 Part your hair on the opposite side

This teeny trick will keep your guy glancing your way all day. He'll know something's *different*. But what? Go ahead and keep him guessing. Haven't you heard that maintaining a little mystery is the ultimate aphrodisiac?

79 Wear fire-engine red

There's a reason why red was picked to paint stop signs: It's one *very* arresting color. Wear a red dress, red shoes, red anything, and it'll make you feel on fire.

80 Button up

Wearing something with lots and lots of buttons may sound like it'll make getting out of your clothes quite a production, but there is an upside: It'll make getting out of your clothes quite a production! Undressing will automatically feel like a striptease as you slowly work your way from clasp to clasp. Or, if he's inspired to free you from your garments himself, the extra time and care it'll take will build the anticipation to bodice-ripping levels.

81 Apply lipstick in front of him

This old-school sexy move is one few men can resist. How could they? After all, you're lavishing attention on your luscious lips.

SURPRISING SEX FACT!

74 percent of women regularly don lingerie to liven things up, according to REDBOOK poll. What's more, 61 percent of men think a woman dressed in lingerie is sexier than one naked.

82   Trade in your sweats for a sexier alternative

Repeat after us: Being comfortable doesn't mean you can't look cute. Even on those days you're just lounging around at home with your guy, resist the urge to reach for anything with an elastic waist band. Instead, opt for a cute T-shirt and tap pants, or a deep V-neck sweater and sexy jeans, which will instantly transform your mood from sluggish vegetable to up-for-anything vixen.

83   Wear leather

We don't care if it's a jacket, skirt, pants, or even just a cuff bracelet. The slightest hint of hide carries a bad-girl, biker-chick chic that'll make his heart zoom. (And if real leather gives you qualms, faux is totally fine, too.)

84   Create some eye-catching cleavage

Try this devastating combo: a push-up bra of dizzying proportions, a low-cut top, and a sparkly necklace that tumbles between your heaving bosom. He won't be able to tear his eyes away.

85   Try on his fragrance for a change

Dab his cologne on a few extra-erogenous zones: cleavage, nape of neck, between thighs. Inhaling his masculine scent all day will serve as a constant reminder of what you could be doing once he appears in the flesh.

86 Put on an animal print

Even the smallest accent—a leopard-print scarf, a zebra thong—will make you feel a little more feral.

87 Get a temporary tattoo

Get a cute little heart on your butt cheek, or a long vine climbing up your inner thigh. You'll be dying to show it off—and when you do, his reaction will be priceless (after all, he doesn't need to know it's temporary!).

88 Slip into a strappy tank top

Bra optional. Then watch him try to keep his eyes off you.

89 Try his clothes on for size

There's something about a woman lounging around in a man's white work shirt. Is it the stark contrast of a crisp, starched collar against bare skin? The fact that you're enticingly

SURPRISING SEX FACT!

In a study conducted by the Kinsey Institute and the Olfactory Research Fund, women who caught a whiff of a men's fragrance (Drakkar Noir, to be exact) while fantasizing about an erotic experience reported being more aroused than when exposed to no odor or even a feminine perfume.

marking your territory? The way that, when open except for one strategically located button, the material skims thighs and covers the bare minimum of what needs covering and no more? We don't know, and frankly, we don't care. All we know is, it works!

90 Wear fishnet stockings under your jeans

Even if they're barely peaking out at the ankles, they'll make you feel like a total vamp.

91 Surprise him with a garter belt

Haven't worn one since your wedding? Then it's time to give him a second viewing. (It'll transform you into a sultry femme fatale from a forties movie; perhaps he'll want to role-play the hard-boiled private eye.) On your next night out, slide your guy's palm under your skirt just high enough so that he comes across your little surprise. A sexy mystery will begin!

92 Swipe on some flavored lip gloss

Just knowing that your lips taste like raspberry, watermelon, or passion fruit will have you yearning to plant one on your guy and make him guess the flavor.

93 Trim your bikini line just a little bit more than usual . . .

Trust us, he *will* notice.

> ### *Girl talk tip-off*
>
> "Right after I got a Brazilian this summer, I had this frenzied, crazy sex with my husband, which ended in our having our first-ever simultaneous orgasms! I guess it was the friction or something. Afterward, we both wanted to send my waxer flowers!"
>
> —Alex, 35

94   . . . Or go completely bare down there

Head to a salon and ask for a full Brazilian bikini wax, which will leave you completely bare below the belt. For starters, that smooth sensation south of the border will get you wondering, *Hmm, what would it feel like now if he did*_____[fill in the blank] *to me in bed tonight?* Plus, once he gets a gander, he'll be dying to find out for himself.

95   Smooth on a rich body lotion

Take your sweet time covering every inch of your body with moisturizer. It'll make your skin feel fantastic, and tempt you to show your guy just how soft it is.

96   Wear a candy necklace one night

To get him nibbling, tell him it's his dessert.

97   Untame your mane

Every once in awhile, don't bother blow-drying or styling your hair. Your slightly tousled tresses may tease out a little more of your wild side.

98 Get a silky, nude bra

This material and shade hides, well, *nothing*. Wear under a white T-shirt and he'll wonder *Whoa . . . is she not wearing a bra today?* and get him dying to find out the truth.

99 Skip the underwear

Panty lines: Who needs 'em? And talk about an instant rush: Whether you tell your guy you're going commando or keep this secret all to yourself, it's bound to make the evening more interesting.

100 Wear heels—and nothing else

When getting undressed one evening, take off everything but your stilettos. Casually walk around as if you just haven't bothered to kick them off yet and see how long it takes him to pounce.

101 Slip into something comfortable

We know, full-length silk slips faded from women's wardrobes back in the 1940s. Here's why we should bring 'em back: First, they feel

---

Moves men love

"One night my wife and I were out to dinner and we were sitting at a table, but she wouldn't take off her coat. I asked her why and she said she couldn't—and just stared at me. Turns out, all she was wearing was a trench coat and high heels. I couldn't even eat; all I could think was, 'This is the sexiest thing I've ever seen.'"

—Tom, 31

amazing under whatever you're wearing. Second, they *look* amazing in an Elizabeth Taylor, *Cat on a Hot Tin Roof* kind of way. Make sure it's the first thing he sees you put on in the morning—and the last thing you peel off come nighttime—to spark some Old Hollywood-style romance and feel like a silver screen siren.

102 Break out the bling-bling

Wear nothing but jewelry to bed—it'll fulfill his Vegas-showgirl fantasy. Graze the nape of his neck with your chandelier earrings. Slip on a bunch of bangles and create a clamor under the comforter. Or skim your super long strand of faux pearls up and down his legs. (Earn bonus points if you tie him to the bedpost with them.)

103 Do it dressed

Sometimes, it doesn't matter what you wear, as long as you keep wearing it! Just hike up, pull down, or yank aside any articles of clothing that are in your way. It'll lend a must-have-you-now sizzle to sex that's undeniably hot, hot, hot.

Moves men love

"Some women quit being sexy for their man after they get married, but Nancy has never stopped showing me how hot she is. She has this special walk that's just for me, where she slowly struts around, with her hips swaying from side to side. When she comes home from work, she keeps the high heels on for 10 or 15 minutes—long enough so that she knows I'm getting an eyeful of that sexy walk. I want to take her straight to the bedroom."

—Mark, 32

CHAPTER 6

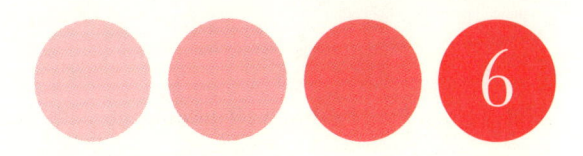

Get your sexercise!

It's a scientific fact: Women who work up a sweat have hotter sex. And no, it's not because they're sporting six-pack abs or a size-four butt. It's because exercise gives them more energy, better flexibility, improved circulation, and other benefits that pay off big-time once they hit the sheets. Which workouts are best? We're glad you asked. Consider the exercises below your own personal boot camp to get your sex life in tip-top shape. Unlike the usual ways to work up a sweat, these routines target parts of your anatomy that *really* come into play when you're getting it on (and we bet your personal trainer won't teach these things, either). What's more, many of these activities can be done in your home, no gym or jogging bra required. In other words, you have no excuse—and once you feel the Olympic-level impact in bed, you won't want one. Ten-hut!

104   The Cat Stretch

The benefit: It's simple: The more flexible you are *out* of bed, the more flexible you'll be *in* bed—and the greater your ability to contort in all sorts of sex positions (and we've got plenty of suggestions along those lines in chapter 17).

How to do it: Get on all fours, with your hands directly underneath your shoulders and your knees directly beneath your hips. Inhale deeply and arch your back, elongating your spine from the top of your neck to your tailbone. Look upward slightly. Then exhale and tuck in your tailbone, dropping your head and pressing the middle of your spine up toward the ceiling. Repeat 10 times for better flex—and better sex.

105   The Hot Hips Swivel

The benefit: More fluid hip movements, which are bound to come in handy once you get horizontal.

How to do it: Stand with your feet apart, your knees slightly bent, and with your hands on your waist. Swivel your hips to the right, front, left, and back, making a smooth counterclockwise circle. After a dozen, reverse direction.

106   The Spinal Stretch

The benefit: People often store tension in their lower back, and that can throw a wrench in the old bump 'n' grind. Loosening the muscles in this area can help.

How to do it: Take a waist-height kitchen stool (ideally with a cushioned seat or pillow on top), lay your upper back on the seat, and let your lower back and pelvis hang free. Reaching your arms overhead for balance, you should feel the muscles in your lower back relax. Breathe deeply. Work your way up to stretching like this for five minutes at a time.

107 The Diaphragm Flexor

The benefit: Strange but true: Many women don't breathe properly during sex. Rather than inhaling deeply, they pant in shallow bursts, which denies their body of the oxygen it needs to get fully aroused. To change this habit, you need to strengthen your diaphragm, the muscles located beneath your lungs and above your abdomen.

How to do it: Breathe in slowly so that your stomach expands, keeping your shoulders and ribcage as motionless as possible. Then, exhale slowly, feeling your stomach contract. First try this exercise on your own to get a feel for it, then try to consciously incorporate it during sex—the added O_2 boost should make a difference.

108 The Quadriceps Crunch

The benefit: The muscles on the front of your thighs are the powerhouse behind most woman-on-top sex positions. Keep them toned and you'll never tire of this take-charge pose.

How to do it: Try the "wall sit," where you lean your back against a wall and then slide down so your thighs are parallel to the floor. Hold this position for 30 seconds, building up to one or two minutes at a time.

109 The Head-to-Toe Tingler

The benefit: This exercise will improve circulation from head to toe and boost your energy levels—a perfect warm-up before you pounce on him.

How to do it: Get down on all fours. Keeping your butt lifted, walk your hands forward until your head and chest are near the floor. Tilt your pelvis so your butt goes up even higher, then tilt back down. Continue rocking your pelvis up and down for up to one minute. Next, thrust your body forward and up, shifting your weight onto your hands. (Your body should be nearly straight from shoulders to knees, and your arms should be straight, with your shoulders above your hands.) As you lean forward, inhale and gently squeeze your buttocks together. Now exhale and push back to your original position (weight on knees, butt in the air). Repeat for up to one minute.

110 The Pink Flamingo

The benefit: This is a great cardio workout that also increases flexibility in your inner thighs, a definite advantage for many sex positions.

How to do it: Pick out tunes that make you want to move, and dance to the music any way you want—but add kicks, as high and as often as you can kick. If you don't exercise much, start with low, gentle kicks and build up slowly to avoid injury. Do this for at least 5 minutes, building up to 15 on the days you have time for a longer workout.

111 The Classic Kegel

The benefit: Kegel exercises (you've probably heard of them) are a cornerstone to sexual fitness, and here's why: They tone your pubococcygeal (PC) muscles, which encircle your vaginal opening and contract rhythmically during orgasm. The stronger your PC muscles, the stronger your orgasm. And the stronger your orgasm, the bigger the smile on your face afterward, of course!

How to do it: First off, make sure you know which muscles we're talking about (you can locate the PC muscle by stopping and starting the flow of urine). Slowly contract your PC muscles and hold for three seconds. Then relax and repeat, working your way up to 25 or 30 reps per session.

112 The Flutter Kegel

The benefit: Think of it as interval training: A variation on the Classic Kegel, this workout gives you increased control over these key muscles, which can further enhance blood flow and sexual responsiveness when you get randy.

How to do it: Squeeze and relax these muscles in regular, rapid succession for ten seconds, building up to 15- or 20-second time periods as you get a hang of it.

SURPRISING SEX FACT!

Just 20 minutes of upping your heart rate instantly increases testosterone levels and sexual responsiveness, according to a study from the University of British Columbia, Canada

113 The Downward Kegel

The benefit: While regular Kegels work out the muscles that contract in the upward motion, this exercise hits those oft-ignored muscles that come into play in the downward direction.

How to do it: During regular Kegels, as you relax gently bear down or push out for a beat before contracting again.

Plus: 5 regular workouts with sexy benefits

114 Sit-ups

When you do stomach crunches, your pelvic muscles, which support your reproductive organs and contract during orgasm, also get toned. And the stronger those muscles are, the more intense your climax will be.

115 Pilates

This system of core-strengthening exercises can pump up the pelvic floor muscles. The more control and awareness you have over them, the greater the sensitivity in that area, and the sweeter sex will feel.

116 Power walking

Doing laps around your neighborhood improves blood flow to your entire body, including areas below the belt. To reap the bedroom benefits, aim for at least 20 minutes of aerobic activity three to four times a week.

117 Skating

Hitting the rink strengthens your inner thighs, a typically weak area for women. Tone these muscles and you'll find that when you squeeze them together during intercourse, you'll both get a snugger fit—a plus for him and you.

118 Yoga

Flexibility *and* focus improve, making it easier to turn off the never-ending to-do list in your brain ("I'm out of dog food!" "The dryer needs unloading!") and fully devote your mind and body to that sexy guy next to you.

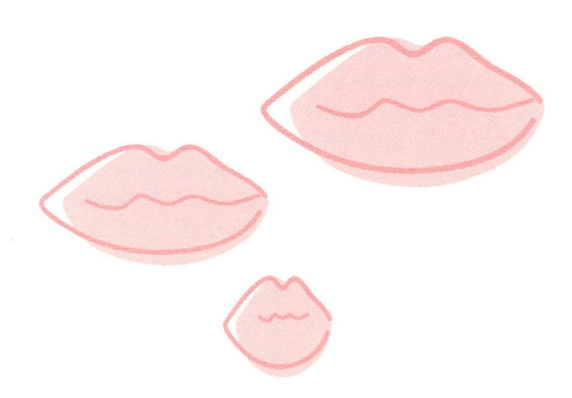

chapter 7

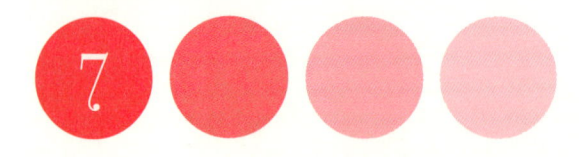

Eat your way to better sex

No doubt about it, eating is fun. So much fun, in fact, that you're probably tempted to head to the fridge right now and inhale that leftover pasta or pint of Häagen-Dazs calling your name. But what, you might be wondering, does this have to do with sex? Believe it or not, plenty. Studies show that certain vitamins and minerals can boost hormone levels, increase nerve sensitivity, and make sex sizzle in all sorts of subtle yet noticeable ways. The next time you're wondering why you're feeling so amorous over dinner, see if one of these foods below may be to blame . . . and maybe you'll want to give it a permanent spot on your grocery list. Bon appétit!

119   Caviar

This delicious delicacy has more than fancy cocktail party cachet going for it. Fish eggs are rich in magnesium, a mineral that helps increase sexual stamina and sensitivity. So, don't be surprised if the hanky-panky you have later on really hits the spot.

120   Chocolate

There's a reason this cocoa confection is the drug of choice for the majority of womankind. It contains a compound called methylxanthine, which triggers the release of dopamine in the body. This, in turn, can leave you woozy with pleasure and make you melt in his arms.

121   Coffee

Sure, your Starbucks habit may keep you from snoozing at your office, but caffeine has other perks too, like the ability to heighten sensations, sexual and otherwise. So, when in doubt, make that single espresso a double!

122   Eggs

Hard-boiled, scrambled, sunny-side up, down, or sideways, eggs are full of vitamin B6, which help your body balance hormone levels and cope with stress. Is your psycho boss or mother-in-law cramping your lovemaking mojo? Order an omelet to set things right, or try other foods that are rich in B6 (spinach, carrots, peas, sunflower seeds, wheat germ, or fish).

123 French fries

No, they're not great for your cholesterol levels. But potatoes contain vitamin B5, and vitamin B5 is essential for the production of sex hormones, and sex hormones are essential for making us chase each other around like crazed maniacs. Talk about a sexy chain reaction.

124 Garlic

Granted, your breath is a veritable weapon of mass destruction for hours afterward, but get past that minor downside, and this pungent seasoning will spice up your sex life by dilating blood vessels and improving circulation throughout your nether regions.

125 Ginger

Whether you take it in tea or on top of your sushi, this Eastern relish revs your metabolism, which can get your whole body humming with renewed sexual energy.

126 Ginkgo biloba tea

Brew a pot and teatime might turn into for-two time. According to studies, this herb will get your blood pumping due south, straight to your genitals.

127 Honey

Take sugar in your tea? Switch to this gooey alternative. It contains boron, a mineral that can increase your body's levels of the libido-boosting hormone testosterone.

128 Milk

Calcium isn't just good for your teeth and bones, it's also a must for your muscles—including those that contract during orgasm. If you're not a dairy drinker, you can also get this nutrient from broccoli and sweet potatoes.

129 Oatmeal

This breakfast cereal might not *look* sexy, but studies show that oats increase testosterone levels in your blood (morning sex, anyone?).

130 Oranges

Foods high in vitamin C don't just fight colds, they also may prompt a tumble or two. That's because vitamin C ups your body's levels of oxytocin, a hormone that encourages you to bond in the most straightforward way we humans know—by cuddling.

131 Oysters

This oft-joked-about aphrodisiac is one that actually lives up to its legendary status, and no, it's not only because they look like, well, use your imagination here. It's because they're loaded with zinc and other minerals that serve as the building blocks for sex hormones—and since these substances are already in salt form, they're instantly usable by the body. So get ready . . . slurp . . . strip!

132 Soy

Soy burgers, soy sauce—it's all good, since tofu binds with estrogen receptors, thereby boosting sexual responsiveness. Studies also show this little legume combats symptoms of menopause—particularly hot flashes—and can benefit your guy as well by improving the health of his prostate, a sex organ that's involved in the production of semen.

133 Steak

Carnivores rejoice! Beef and dark-meat poultry can help curb the body's production of prolactin, a hormone that at high levels can dampen your doing-it drive. Don't worry, veggie lovers, you can get the same passion-pumping perks from brown rice, whole-brain bread, green leafy vegetables, and crumbly cheeses like Cheshire or Lancashire.

134 Strawberries

Sure, these plump, cute little berries are pretty sexy-looking already. But on top of that, they contain antioxidants and improve circulation, which up your chances of having a hot-blooded encounter.

135 Sushi

Order a roll, and you'll get a double-whammy libido lift. First off, fatty fish like tuna and salmon are high in omega-3 and L-arginine, substances that stir sexual arousal. Second, the seaweed wrapping is packed with iodine, an ingredient that improves thyroid function and keeps your lovemaking motor running smoothly (in fact, women suffering from low sex drive often have a mild case of hypothyroidism, say experts).

136 Tabasco sauce

This heady concoction inflames more than your taste buds. One of its main ingredients, chili peppers, contains capsaicin, a chemical that triggers changes in your body that mimic sexual arousal. Just think: A mere sprinkle on your burrito makes you feel flushed, sweaty, and your heart races. Why not take advantage of your heightened state and reach for your guy instead of a glass of water?

137 Walnuts

This snack is chock-full of fatty acids, which are a major component in sex hormones. So go ahead and toss some on your salad or in your brownie mix to get your sexy back by tonight.

138 Wine

Okay, so we all know booze can lower your inhibitions and lead to all sorts of mayhem. But alcohol also contains estradiol, a substance that, in women, is linked to increased lubrication and libido. Just beware, *too* much imbibing depresses your nervous system and makes you crave sleep rather than sex.

Plus: 4 infamous "aphrodisiacs" to avoid

139 Horny-goat weed

So named by an ancient goat herder who noticed his flock got frisky after grazing on it. But the sexual powers of this plant (also known as epimedium) are dubious at best, say experts.

140 Kava

This Pacific island plant may lull you into a more amorous mood, but it's banned or restricted in six countries because it can cause liver problems. Worth it? We think not.

141 Spanish fly

Perhaps the most well-known aphrodisiac, it's also the most deadly. Extracted from a blister beetle (why it's called a fly, we have no clue), even a tiny dose can cause kidney failure, heart attack, and stroke.

142 Yohimbe

This tree bark is purported to improve blood flow to the genitals. While studies support this claim, talk to your doctor before trying it. It can be dangerous for people with high blood pressure.

> **SURPRISING SEX FACT!**
>
> In one study, people who took a vitamin C supplement had sex 68 percent more often than the sorry subjects popping a placebo.

CHAPTER 8

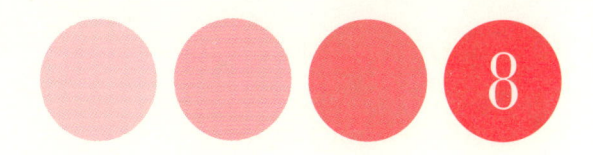

Got a hot date?

Finally! You've got a date. Sure, maybe it's with a guy who, at this point, sees you slathered in a face mask every night and buys you tampons. But still, a date is a date, and even if your courting days are over that doesn't mean your evening together should end with a good-night hug (laaame!). Whether you're going out to a movie or staying in to take a crack at making paella, the very best dates, of course, are merely long, delicious lead-ups to getting things cooking with each other, right? To help that happen, we've put together some ideas on how to make your rendezvous feel as sexually charged as when you two first met and, we hope, make your date last way past your bedtime.

Going out? Then try these ideas...

143 Let him pick out what you wear

You make so many decisions all day, every day. Why not give yourself one less thing to think about—and give him something fun to do in the process? Before a night out, step out of the shower and throw in the towel, so to speak. Let him pick out your skirt, top, shoes, lipstick, panties, perfume, everything. What he chooses may surprise you, and nothing's hotter than a surprise between two people who think they know everything about each other.

144 Return to the source

That restaurant where you exchanged your first awkward so-what-do-you-dos, that street corner where he first laid his lips on yours are perfect places to rediscover if you want to bring back a rush of those initial in-love feelings—and more.

145 Play a bar game

Darts? Foosball? Scrabble? Anything will do. Then tell him you want to make things interesting with a sexy wager: Whoever loses has to_____ [fill in the blank—and make it good].

146 Order a piña colada

One sip of this pineapple-and-coconut cocktail will transport you to a mental place filled with sparkling sand, seminaked bodies, and (of course) lots 'n' lots of vacation sex. Want to make it a trip for two? Ask for an extra straw and tempt him to partake.

147 Order food that'll fire things up

Believe it or not, what you pick off a menu can impact your hanky-panky potential later—and spicy food, by far, delivers the biggest passion punch. The reason: That flushed, sweaty feeling brought on by lamb vindaloo or Szechuan spicy beef revs your metabolism, which can lift even the most sluggish libido from its postdinner lull and keep you feeling feisty rather than full.

148 Ban all mention of nonsexy subjects

At home, everything from his hemorrhoids to that home-repair project is fair game. But on a date, the banter should feel like an escape from life's mundane concerns. So, feel free to meander down memory lane ("What would you say was our best vacation ever?") or frolic in wish-fulfillment territory ("If you could blink your eyes and be anywhere, where would we be?"), but if it's something you *need* to say (other than "I want you—now"), save it for one of the other 23 hours of your day.

149 Look into his eyes while you eat dessert

Decadent dishes like tiramisu aren't meant to be wolfed down like a burger and fries. Instead, take your time to savor each bite while you gaze into his eyes and show him just how much you're enjoying it. Trust us, it's a sexy sight, so much so that neighboring tables may pull a *When Harry Met Sally* and tell their server, "I'll have what she's having."

150   Mimic his movements

If his legs are crossed, cross yours. If he's leaning forward with his chin in his hands, do the same. If he smiles, grin right back. This technique, which scientists call "mirroring," builds rapport by signaling that you two are perfectly in sync . . . and primed to link up in a much more literal way once you finish your last bites in unison and get the heck outta there.

151   Shake your thang

There's a reason why dancing is a date-night staple: It naturally enacts the "mirroring" principal described in the previous tip. Be it swing, salsa, or just the two of you swaying to the sounds of a jukebox, a little dancing all but guarantees that by the end of the night, you will be doing the horizontal mambo.

152   Take advantage of long tablecloths

Out at a restaurant that offers good coverage below the waist? Between courses, let your fingers wander over to your man's lap or bring his hand over to your own. A few sweet (or saucy) strokes, and he'll be asking the waiter for a to-go bag in no time.

> > Inside the male mind

"When we're at a dinner party and she's in the mood for some privacy with me, she'll take my hand under the table and place it on her leg—and then push it up dangerously high on her thigh. Instantly, I can't think of anything except getting home with her as fast as possible."

—Paul, 38

153   Play footsie

This seductive move is so "classic it's a cliché" for a reason: It's fun! You can do it in the middle of a restaurant or dinner party with no one knowing, which makes it your sexy little secret. Need a little footsie refresher course? Drop your shoe and let your bare foot travel up his leg and swirl circles around his calf muscle. Then swoop back down and give his ankle a taste of the action. If he starts stuttering, that's a good sign. Smile a mischievous smile and repeat.

154   Watch a scary movie

Not only does a frightening flick prompt lots of hand-squeezing and lap-jumping, it floods your body with adrenaline, which makes you more alert—and aroused. It's instinctual: When our ancestors felt their lives were threatened for real by, say, a saber-toothed tiger, it triggered an urge to fight, flee, and (once the crisis was over, of course) procreate. Trip those primordial alarm bells yourself, and it might be just the jolt you need to get busy.

155   Rev up your hand-holding

Remember back in the day when the feel of his hand on yours made your stomach flip? The next time you're out at the movies, let him know you've got more than Tom Hanks' latest blockbuster in mind by running your fingers up and down his arm or interlacing your fingers with his and tracing circles on his palm with your thumb. Sweet, but also suggestive of what's in store after the closing credits roll.

156 Check out some X-rated art

Skim the art reviews in your local paper for exhibits that sound sexually provocative (some classic options to keep an eye out for: the amorous nudes of Auguste Rodin, Japanese *shunga*, or ancient Greek pottery, which is often carved with couplings, triplings, and more). Since it's art, you can discuss what you see without feeling sleazy, and yet also get your gears turning ("Look, we've never tried *that* before, have we?").

157 Shoot him a coy, come-hither glance

The next time your honey tears himself away from your side to fetch a drink for you at the bar or to say hello to a coworker who happens to be sitting nearby, make the most of your time apart by checking him out as if he were a stranger. Here's how: From across the room, catch his eye and hold it for just a beat, then look away. Then glance back quickly, shyly, out of the corner of your eye, letting your gaze flicker up and down his body. He'll be back at your side before you know it.

Moves men love

"My wife, Laura, plays a world-class game of footsie. She has beautiful feet and wears a lot of high heels. She runs the side of her foot up and down my calf, first on the outside of my leg, then the inside. Then she kicks off her shoes and caresses my legs with her bare feet. Her toes tickle my ankles. If we're at home or sitting in the dark back booth of our favorite neighborhood pub, she puts her bare feet in my lap, and...I can't stand up for a while afterward."

—Bill, 37

>> Inside the male mind

"While we were at the movies, she took my hand from around her shoulder and placed it against her breast. Then she started gently caressing my hand with hers. This move was so simple and passionate that I had sex on my mind until the movie ended. Her seductive gesture allowed the anticipation to build to incredible heights that night."

—Tom, 35

158 Make your hearts race—literally

Take a joint tennis lesson, hike up a mountain trail, or hit the road for a three-mile run. The physical exhilaration begets *more* physical exhilaration—just wait until you get home, jump in the shower, and take advantage of that adrenaline rush in other ways.

159 Seduce via stemware

At dinner, run your fingers up and down, up and down the stem of his wineglass. Take a seductive sip from it and slowly lick your lips while staring into his eyes. By laying claim to his property, you're giving him permission to lay claim to you, too.

160 Canoodle like the celebs

Who says you have to be a Hollywood "It" girl to get caught sneaking a sensuous snuggle with your man? The next time you're dining *à deux*, squeeze in next to him on the same side of the booth or table, as if you're at the most romantic café in Paris. Then let your tongue do the talking.

Moves men love

"Recently my sweetheart got me a gift certificate to Victoria's Secret. She said, 'Let's go shopping—and you can buy anything you want me to wear.' Being allowed to call the shots on the purchases we made was an amazing turn-on. That shopping spree was one long stretch of foreplay!"

—Tyson, 28

161 Take a walk together in the rain

Snuggle under the umbrella together or, if it's only sprinkling, brave the elements without one. Your rain-kissed look will definitely get him hankering to get you out of those wet clothes.

162 Stroll to the ice cream parlor

Sure, it *sounds* innocent. But not if you get a cone instead of a cup, and take your sweet time licking the sides while looking straight at him (a glint in your eye can't hurt, either).

163 Go on a sexy shopping spree

Head to your favorite lingerie store and ask him to pick out something for you to try on . . . then give him a sneak peek in the dressing room.

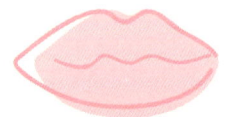

164 Get dressed to the nines

Then, just as you're about to head out the door, make yourselves late. What better way is there to kick off the evening and (nudge nudge, wink wink) inspire more shenanigans later?

Staying in? Then try these ideas . . .

165 Whip up a spread of finger fare

Sure, silverware is the civilized way to go, but civilized isn't exactly sexy, now is it? So, skip the utensils one evening and stick with bite-size morsels of sushi, chicken skewers, or a cheese-and-fruit plate. You'll feel like Greek gods as you languidly lick your fingers between bites and slip grapes into each other's mouth.

166 Throw an impromptu picnic

Ditch your oh-so-formal kitchen table and lay down a blanket on your living room floor or (weather permitting) in your backyard. Dining while reclining is inherently more make-out worthy; prepare for some not-so-innocent necking to take place.

> > Inside the male mind

"I don't know what it is, but watching my wife sucking on an ice pop or licking an ice cream cone makes me so crazy. Maybe it's the thought of how else she can apply those skills."

—Matthew, 29

167 — Get him to really focus on the food

Break out the blindfolds or just have your husband close his eyes while you feed him treats, such as mango slices or a decadent spoonful of Nutella, à la *9 1/2 Weeks*. This will get him to hone in on sensations he normally takes for granted—and make your usual at-home dinner feel a whole lot edgier.

168 — Play a sensual soundtrack

Music is the ultimate mood-altering substance, so burn a CD or make an iMix featuring your favorites. Need some suggestions? Try "Tonight Is the Night" by Betty Wright, "Naughty Girl" by Beyoncé, or the slow, sultry tunes of Diana Krall, Lucinda Williams, or Norah Jones to pump up the passion.

Moves men love

"We were at a museum for a black-tie event, and I was feeling sharp with my wife on my arm. As we looked at a painting, she subtly brushed one of her breasts against my arm. At the next painting, she did it again—and yet again when we were in front of a sculpture. At this point we were both suppressing giggles because the well-heeled crowd was clueless about our devious behavior, which made her sneaky seduction even hotter. Finally, we ducked into an empty gallery room for a quick kiss, then took the shortest route possible to get our coats."

—Bill, 41

One woman's sex secret—revealed

"During our honeymoon, my husband and I had awesome sex to Prince. Now when we hear it, we both get that sly twinkle in our eyes. To make sure we do it often, one of us will play it as a clear sign that we're about to, um, make music together. It's kept our marriage just as passionate as it was when we first tied the knot."

—Rachel, 33

169 Slow dance

Face it, there's something unbelievably intimate about snuggling hip to hip and rocking from side to side—especially if you do it at home where no one's watching. What's to stop you from letting your hands wander?

170 Rent a chick flick

Of course, we know pretty much any romantic comedy with John Cusack or Hugh Grant will get *you* feeling lovey-dovey. But as much as guys are loath to admit it, these movies work magic on them, too. Case in point: In one study by the University of Michigan, men who viewed a romantic scene from *The Bridges of Madison County* experienced a boost in their levels of progesterone, a hormone that helps people bond. The moral of the story: If you want to get your way in the movie-picking date-night debate, inform him that chick flicks are scientifically proven to get him (yes, him) in the mood for some nuzzling—and you'll be right there with him.

> ### Moves men love
>
> *"She loves to shave my beard before we make love. It's so intimate and sensual having her body so close to mine as she runs the razor over my face. Plus, there's something so nurturing about it; we always end up all over each other afterward."*
>
> —Mike, 36

171 Engage in mutual grooming

You shave his beard; he paints your toenails. You draw a bath and loofah his back; he gives you a slow, sensual hair washing. It's instinctual: Animals often tidy each other up before pairing off; consider this your own version of fluffing feathers and rooting for fleas before you go a-mating. Not only does it get you looking your best, it makes you both feel cared for, which is the ultimate aphrodisiac for every life form from ladybugs on up to little old you.

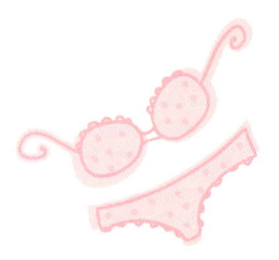

> ### Moves men love
>
> *"She turns up the stereo really, really loud, she grabs me, and we dance around the house together. We have a favorite Sinatra CD that's always ready to go full blast!"*
>
> —Sean, 30

172 Use fondue as foreplay

No doubt about it, this gooey food oozes groovy come-and-get-me vibes. Don't worry if it gets a little messy—licking sticky fingers (his or your own) is kinda the point.

173 Try erotic aromatherapy

Light a scented candle that reminds you of a past time and place where you two got it on, and how. Research has shown that your sense of smell is strongly associated with your memories, so if you and your honey had a romantic weekend at a cabin in the woods, a pine-scented candle will bring it all back, and then some.

174 Stage a private drive-in

Watch a sexy film on the portable DVD player in the car (flicks like *Unfaithful* or even *Wild Things*). Bring lots of popcorn . . . and be sure to steam up the windows.

Girl talk tip-off

"Bathing and washing each other's hair is a great way to get in the mood, since you feel pampered. It's a gentle kind of giving."

—Dina, 30

175 Crack a beer in bed

Pop a few exotic microbrews in the sack, and then drink to the rowdy fun to come. Or, if martinis are more your style, make 'em dirty with extra olive juice.

176 Share a bedtime story

Buy a book of erotica (browse at cleispress.com) and have him read you a story. Hearing his voice describing the sex other people are having can be amazingly arousing. And soon enough, you may find yourself saying, "We should do what they're doing."

177 Take a bubble bath together

Candles lit, him in back, you in front, lotsa bubbles . . . need we say more?

One woman's sex secret—revealed

"My husband and I will flip on Sex and the City *and play 'red light, green light'; we can get hot and heavy only when the couples on screen do. When they're not getting it on, all we can do is lie really close to each other. This allows the tension to build until we're both ready to let loose."*

—Tara, 39

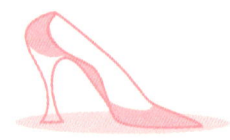

Moves men love

"She'll light candles in the bedroom and pour us each a Scotch on the rocks. Then we sip the drinks in bed and talk before we make love. The experience makes me feel very Cary Grant."

—Ben, 30

178 Play strip Monopoly

Lose a hotel = lose your undies.

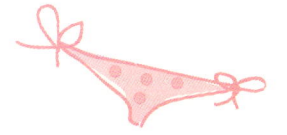

179 Turn TV time into more of a turn-on

Ever heard of those drinking games where, say, everyone takes a swig when a certain TV character flaunts a signature quirk? You can do the same with your sex life: While watching, say, Conan O'Brien, agree to make out every time he licks his lips (which happens a lot). Then, agree to get even friskier every time he spins in a circle. Finally, vow to get it on every time Conan cracks a political joke. Now, who said late-night TV is bad for your sex life?

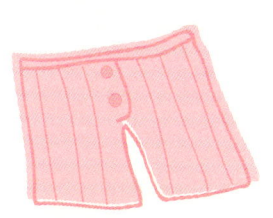

> ### Moves men love
>
> *"One night I was in the living room and my wife called me. As I walked down the hallway, I noticed a line of Hershey's Chocolate Kisses leading into the master bedroom, ending in an arrow pointing toward the bed. It was obvious she wanted to give me more than just kisses that night."*
>
> —Preston, 45

180 Drop a huge hint about what's in store

Whatever you've got planned, drive him crazy with anticipation beforehand by hitting him with this: "I made plans for us on Saturday night. But all I'm telling you is that a bubble bath/Monopoly board/pitcher of margaritas is involved." Just flash a sly smile and keep your lips zipped no matter how hard he tries to tickle the details out of you. The mystery will get him filling in the blanks in all sorts of delicious ways he'll be happy to make good on once the big night arrives.

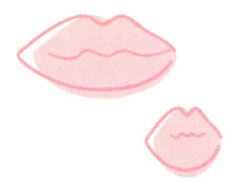

> ### Moves men love
>
> *"Once when I arrived home, I saw a trail of roses leading to the bedroom. There, I found her waiting for me in bed with a smile that could only mean 'Come and get me!'"*
>
> —John, 31

CHAPTER 9

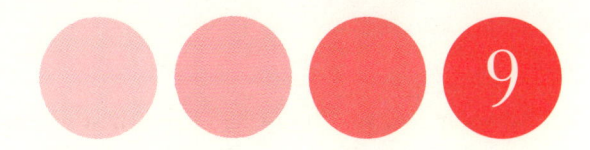

Ladies, make your move!

It's simple, really: If you're craving a cheeseburger, you order it. If you want a promotion, you march into your boss's office and explain why you deserve it. If you want your guy to fix the boiler, you ask him to do it (nicely at first, not-so-nicely the longer it sits unfixed). These days, we gals know that if we want something, the best way to get it is to ask. And yet when it comes to sex, strangely, many of us mentally backpedal about 50 years and think, Well, it's the man's job to put the moves on me. Right?

Wrong. The honest truth is, your guy would love, love, love for you to show in no uncertain terms that you're jonesing for him as much as he is for you. But if you're on the bashful side, how do you step up to the plate without feeling so, well, forward? Allow us to help. Here are some moves that even the shyest wallflower can pull off, as well as a few bolder ideas for you daredevils out there. Once you realize what a rush it is to take charge and do the seducing, you'll wonder, What the heck took me so long? Hey, better late than never, right?

181 Give him a wake-up to remember

Wake up and say, "I just had the dirtiest dream." When he asks what it was, insist on showing him.

182 Join him in the shower

"Accidentally" drop the soap and graze every inch of his body on the way down to get it . . . and on the way back up, too, just to make sure he hears loud and clear that lathering up is the least of your concerns.

183 Pencil in some playtime

Surreptitiously snag his day planner and on the date and time of your choice, write "8 p.m.: you + me, alone, in bed." Finally, a meeting he can look forward to!

184 Take off his tie as soon as he's home from work

And his shirt. And his belt. And his pants. And his—you get the idea. And so will he.

SURPRISING SEX FACT!

According to a REDBOOK survey, 55 percent of men say that the number one thing they wish the women in their lives would do more often is initiate sex. So what are you waiting for?

>> Inside the male mind

"I know I'm in for quite a morning when she kisses me awake. The fact that she can't wait until I wake up on my own before pouncing shows me just how much she wants me. This impulsiveness is such a turn-on that I walk on air for the rest of the day."

—Sam, 25

185 Predict his future

The next time you order Chinese takeout, offer to read his fortune cookie for him at the end of the meal. Say, "A very happy ending awaits as soon as you clear the table." (Of course that's not what it *really* says, but you probably won't hear him complaining.)

186 Peruse lingerie sites online together

Browse through some super high-end Web sites, like La Perla (laperla.com) or Agent Provocateur (agentprovocateur.com). Tell him to pick out something outrageously racy he'd like to see you wear one night—then go get it. (Or, if the high-end sticker price makes you feel faint, find something similar but less expensive at Bloomingdale's or Macy's—trust us, he won't notice the difference.)

187 Plant a good-night note

A sure win with dads: Right before he puts the little darlings to sleep, stick a note inside the storybook he's going to read. Tell him *his* bedtime involves some tricks that would put Harry Potter to shame.

Moves men love

"Once when I was putting in long hours at my job, I opened my date planner at work and found a note jotted down on that day's page that said: 'Sex @ 7 p.m.' She must have taken my planner from my briefcase one night and written it in. Needless to say, I was home on time that night!"

—Mike, 42

188 Stage your own *American Idol*

Tell your guy he's judge Simon Cowell and sing him a sassy song. After your performance, tell him you'll do anything—and we mean anything—to stay on the show.

189 Buy some lingerie

Guy lingerie, that is. Get him a pair of silk boxers; set them in a box on the bed with a note saying, "Looking forward to seeing how hot you look in these when I get home tonight."

190 Strip soap-opera style

As soon as you set foot in the front door, start shedding your layers, tossing each article of clothing aside with abandon, leaving a trail to your bed. He'll be hot on your heels.

191 Flop onto the bed and demand that he undress you

Straightforward, effective, and most definitely a command he won't hesitate to obey.

192 Lie in a warm bubble bath

... when you know your hubby's on his way home. Greet him with a soapy, slick foot wave and invite him in, promising it *won't* be just good, clean fun.

193 Bookmark what you want

Want to drop a hot hint of what you're dying to do in bed? Take a copy of *The Joy of Sex*, *The Kama Sutra*, or (shameless plug alert) the book you're reading right now and stick bookmarks on the pages that describe tips you'd like to try. Then leave it where he'll find it.

> ## >> Inside the male mind
>
> *"When I wear button-down shirts, she'll often undo my top two buttons so she can reach in and stroke my chest. Having her undress me puts me completely in her power."*
>
> —Tom, 33

Moves men love

"Sometimes she'll grab my hand and take me to the bedroom. Then she'll lay me down on the bed and have me watch her slowly undress. I love it when she takes charge. Plus, she's usually wearing lingerie under her clothes, which makes me even hotter."

—Michael, 26

194 Be bold

Push him down on the couch and straddle his lap. Pin him against the wall with a kiss as soon as he's walked in the front door. If being aggressive is generally out of character for you, this is all it'll take to make your intentions clear . . . and who knows? You may find it's fun to be a little bossy!

195 Hitch a piggyback ride to bed

Wrap your legs tightly around his waist and bombard him with delicious back-of-the-neck kisses along the way. Then, tell him he deserves a reward for hauling you all the way up there.

SURPRISING SEX FACT!

Not all women are bashful when it comes to getting their guy in bed. According to a REDBOOK survey, 39 percent of women say they initiate sex more often than their husbands do!

196   Charm his pants off

Before he leaves for work, slip a good-luck charm like a penny, four-leaf clover, or rabbit's foot into his pocket with a note saying, "Look who's getting lucky tonight!" Once he comes across this auspicious omen, you can bet your bank account he'll be home early.

197   Shower—but forget the towel

Then call to him to bring you one . . . and ask him to dry you off. Inviting him to put his hands all over your wet, just-washed body will get him thinking anything but clean thoughts.

198   Rip his shirt off

Trust us, there'll be *no* mistaking what's on your mind (and talk about passionate!). Target ratty old button-downs for best results (ripping off a T-shirt is trickier than it looks).

Moves men love

"One morning while I was in the shower, my wife unexpectedly joined me and slowly soaped up my entire body. It was pretty obvious that getting clean wasn't her top priority. I was so aroused I could barely wait to get her into bed."

—Keith, 36

Moves men love

"We were watching a football game, and after the second quarter ended, she said, 'I've got a great idea for halftime.' Then she grabbed my shirt collar and led me to our bed. Seeing her act so flirty and fun about sex reminded me what a vixen she is."

—William, 33

199 Play a sexy version of Hangman

Choose words or phrases that describe things you want to try in bed. Once he figures it out, he'll be all too willing to make those mystery words a reality.

200 Give him a special delivery

Slip a racy magazine in the mailbox with a Post-it that reads, "Thought you might enjoy a little extra reading material." What red-blooded male wouldn't want to share some choice highlights?

>> Inside the male mind

"One afternoon my wife said to me slyly, 'The kids are napping, and I do not have a headache.' This sexy come-on could not have been more clear!"

—Gary, 31

Girl talk tip-off

"We went the classic chocolate-syrup-and-whipped-cream route. The experience was very exciting. Due to the sticky-mess factor, however, I highly recommend saving such antics for hotel visits. You get all the pleasure and none of the cleanup."

—Michelle, 24

201   Send him off with a sexy grocery list

Your must-haves: chocolate sauce, honey, powdered sugar, whipped cream. Call his cell and tell him exactly what you plan on doing with it all—you'll drive him wild right there in aisle nine!

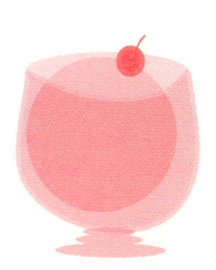

Moves men love

"Every once in a while my wife will surprise me with the best possible gift: an at-home sex date. She'll whisper, 'The kids are staying at the baby-sitter's overnight,' and I'll know exactly what our plans are that evening."

—Anthony, 33

SURPRISING SEX FACT!

57 percent of couples have lathered each other in whipped cream, chocolate, or used some other food during lovemaking, according to a REDBOOK poll.

202 Channel surf your way to sex

Click your way to Cinemax (a.k.a. Skinemax) and linger on one of their scantily-clad late-night flicks until he takes the hint . . . in, oh, about five seconds.

Moves men love

"She got up from the couch, sighed loudly and said she was going to take a nap. She walked away, casually removing her clothes and looking over her shoulder at me. By the time I got to the bedroom, she was lying on the bed naked. She continued to 'sleep' as I began to kiss her. It was like an erotic dream brought to life!"

—Mark, 32

CHAPTER 10

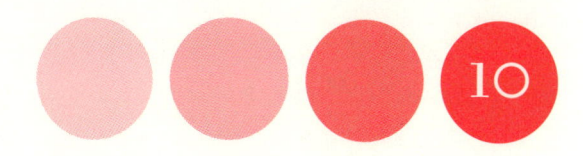

12 totally new kisses to try on your guy

Chances are you know a thing or two about how to lock lips with your guy—after all, smooching was probably the very first trick in your sexual repertoire. Still, are you positive you're pushing your kissing skills to their full potential? Want to be sure? Then allow us to open your eyes to all the amazing mouth-to-mouth maneuvers there are out there to explore. We'll give you step-by-step, lips-on instructions, plus we'll show you a few other areas on the body that would love to be nuzzled, and how. Read on, go find a willing recipient, pucker up, and plant one!

But first, some basic rules to keep in mind...

203 Prep your kisser

It doesn't matter *how* much he loves you, he doesn't love your dragon breath. So, stay smooch-worthy by brushing your teeth *and* your tongue, where much of the bacteria lie (for an extra-fresh kick, try baking soda instead of toothpaste). If you're out, keep mints handy in your purse; gum is fine too, but make sure to get rid of it before you start kissing. If you're caught without breath freshener right when you need it (say, after downing a plate of linguini with garlic sauce), chomp on the sprig of parsley that most restaurants are smart enough to plant on your plate for just such an occasion.

204 Watch the lipstick

Sure, it makes your precious little pout *look* amazing, but it can cause a mess once you two start smacking. What's more, some men aren't crazy about the taste. Flavored lip gloss might be a better alternative, or just ask your man where he stands on the issue so you can doll yourself up accordingly.

SURPRISING SEX FACT!

Americans go lip-to-lip an average of five times every 24 hours, according to a survey of more than 2,200 men and women by Close-Up Tooth-paste. Have you filled your kissing quota for the day?

SURPRISING SEX FACT!

67 percent of men are fine and dandy if you kiss them wearing lipstick, although 25 percent would prefer a makeup-free mouth, and 8 percent actually love getting a taste of flavored lip gloss.

205 Think about what the rest of your body is doing

Remember, your lips are important but hardly the only body part involved in an incredible make-out session. For extra passion points, run your fingers through his hair. Cradle his face in your hands. Stand chest-to-chest so you can feel each other's hearts beating. Squeeze his butt. Maybe you usually kiss with your eyes closed, or, perhaps you prefer keeping your peepers peeled. Either way, try the opposite. You may be pleasantly surprised.

206 Lock lips when he least expects it

Sometimes the most passionate interludes are the ones that occur out of the blue. So go ahead, ambush him with a smooch while you're stuck at a stoplight. Or the next time you're bickering about housework, finances, or some other unsexy topic, stop midsentence, grab him, and go at it. Then pull away, sigh regretfully, and resume the discussion. We guarantee, it'll put your insignificant squabble in perspective and also make him *much* more agreeable.

Now, some totally new kisses to try . . .

207 The Yin-Yang Kiss

Get ready to feel as if you're melting into each other: Take his bottom lip between yours while he takes your top lip between his. Then, start sucking, gently. Once you two have the hang of it, switch so *you're* on top and he's down below, alternating as the mood strikes. This kiss takes teamwork, but that's a good thing—tuning into each other's whims is bound to get you bonding in a whole new way.

208 The Barely-There Kiss

Mouth-to-mouth action isn't the only way to make his knees buckle. A light hint of a smooch near—but not on—his kisser can also work wonders. Starting on his forehead, softly graze your lips over to his temple before slowly swooping down to his mouth. Then, with the tip of your tongue, trace your way around the edges of his lips. At this point, the anticipation will be killing

> ## >> Inside the male mind
>
> *"Aimee is from Paris—and really knows how to French kiss. First, she flirts with my lips in light, teasing, licking kisses. She puts the tip of her tongue into my mouth, quickly pulls it back out, then slides it in again like she's playing hide-and-seek with me in my mouth. She teases my lips again and lightly sucks each one. Then she moves the tip of her tongue in circles just inside my lips. Is that a fire starter? Oh, yeah."*
>
> —Cal, 37

SURPRISING SEX FACT!

According to the book *The Art of Kissing*, by William Cane, 82 percent of would-be canoodlers say the biggest turnoff is bad breath.

him . . . but don't give in just yet. Instead, lean in and lick just the corners of his lips (believe it or not, these two points are potent erogenous zones). From there, it's up to you what happens next—but we guarantee that whatever it is, he'll be raring to go.

209   The Classic French Kiss

Sure, we all know that a French kiss involves some tantalizing tongue action. Here are some sexy ways to add a little *je ne sais quoi* to your technique: Twist your tongue around his in circles. Explore his teeth and gums as if you were searching for something. To make him really jump, flick your tongue across the roof of his mouth (this area can be very ticklish). Master these moves and voilà, you're now worthy of necking on a park bench in Paris.

One woman's sex secret—revealed

"I've kissed my husband thousands of times, but sometimes I'll pretend it's the first time. One morning I kissed him this way as he left for work. He was expecting the usual peck, but instead I went all out. He said, 'Work can wait' before leading me to bed. It's nice to know I can still slay him with a kiss!"

—Barbara, 32

210 French Kiss with a Twist

This is your typical Frenchie (see the previous tip for more details), but here's where things get even *more* interesting: Gently suck on his tongue as it enters your mouth.

211 The Upside-Down Kiss

> **SURPRISING SEX FACT!**
>
> Why do the French get a whole kiss to their credit, anyhow? In 1923, the term "French kiss" was coined as a slur against the culture, which was deemed overly obsessed with the good things in life (and the problem is . . . ?). The French, however, don't call it Frenching, but tongue kissing or soul kissing.

Tobey Maguire and Kirsten Dunst made this smooch famous in the *Spiderman* films, and there's a very good reason this smacker was such a blockbuster: Kissing upside down feels *completely* different than it does right side up. To do it, have him lean back on the arm of a couch while you move in so your eyes are over his chin and your top lip's aligned with his bottom one. Then give him some sugar and judge for yourself.

212 The Neck Nibble

Few kisses pack more passion than those on the neck—but what you might not know is that certain areas are better to nuzzle than others. To make sure you're hitting his main drag, gently pull his head back and to the side, which will expose an extrasensitive tendon running from the ear to the shoulder. Starting at the base of his ear, work your way down the ridge, randomly alternating between small nibbles and gentle kisses so he won't know what's coming next.

>> Inside the male mind

"Kissing is romantic, but having my wife suck on my tongue is so much more of a turn-on. And a guy can't help being reminded of oral sex."

—Tim, 35

213 Déjà-vu Kiss

Close your eyes and imagine you're pressing your lips against his for the very first time. This simple mental shift can bring back a flood of first-kiss electricity.

214 The Guess-That-Flavor Game

Find a flavor he likes, then partake prekiss—eat an orange wedge, sip some hot chocolate, or take a swig of his favorite night cap. Once you start canoodling, he'll probably say, "You taste good, what is that?" Keep kissing until he figures it out.

215 The Hollywood Kiss

Lord knows which Tinseltown twosome first flaunted this rapturous, over-the-top smooch on screen—was it Clark Gable and Vivien Leigh in *Gone With The Wind*? Humphrey Bogart and

SURPRISING SEX FACT!

Two-thirds of men and women close their eyes when they kiss; one-third keep them open.

Ingrid Bergman in *Casablanca*? All we know is that everyone should try it, at least once—better yet, daily. Just have him place his hands on the small of your back and dip you before you lock lips. The fact that you're precariously, breathtakingly draped in his arms may make you swoon like a starlet yourself.

216   The Butterfly Kiss

For this smackeroo, you don't even use your mouth. (After all, who says lips have a monopoly on kissing?) Instead, sidle up to your amour and flutter your eyelashes against his face. Or you can also try it eye-to-eye. Either way, this delicate soupçon of a smooch will feel sublime.

217   The Eskimo Kiss

Take a tip from our frosty friends up north and rub noses rather than going lip to lip. This kiss is sweet, playful, and also a great idea when it's f-f-freezing out and best to keep everything under wraps.

218   The Guinness World Record Kiss

What's the longest you've ever locked lips nonstop? Well, do you want to find out? Go ahead and connect, and when you start feeling breathless, inhale through your nose without breaking your kiss. You can prolong the fun for minutes, hours . . . your call. According to Guinness World Records, the longest kiss ever lasted 30 hours, 59 minutes and 27 seconds, and occurred between Americans Louisa Almedovar and Rich Langley, who took on the challenge in 2001 on *Ricki Lake*. Talk about pucker power!

CHAPTER 11

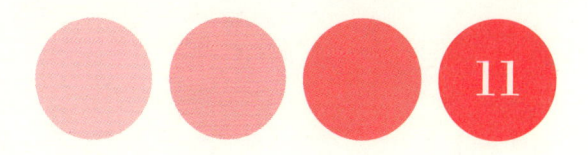

More foreplay, please!

Poor foreplay: relegated to the role of opening act but rarely the main attraction. And yet, as any true sexual connoisseur will tell you, this phase isn't just a tepid warm-up, it's where it's at. Seriously. When else can you devote 100 percent of your efforts to getting in tune with each other's bodies and all but guarantee that what follows next will be more explosive than you'd ever imagined? In other words, it pays to take your sweet time and indulge in the sensual smorgasbord foreplay can be. Here are some fun ways to prolong the agony, hone your skills, and make sure you rub everything (and we mean everything!) the right way.

SURPRISING SEX FACT!

According to a REDBOOK survey, 46 percent of couples spend 3 to 10 minutes on foreplay, while 28 percent linger 10 to 20 minutes; 13 percent of us prolong the agony for more than 20 minutes, while an equal percentage must have a train to catch, since they spend less than 3 minutes on foreplay before moving right along.

219 Play the "How I Like to Be Touched" game

Lie on the bed and have your guy caress you all over, genitals excluded. Have him try different strokes—deep kneading, long slow petting, feathery fondling, and everything in between, to get a gauge of what you like best and where. Take turns, switching off after every 15 to 20 minutes. Ask each other questions like, "Do you like it harder or softer? In circular strokes or when I go up and down?" You may both be surprised just how good an inner-arm tickle or scalp massage feels—and while they might not feel sexual per se, honestly, why quibble about that sort of technicality when it feels so good?

220 Take your sweet time taking his clothes off

If mere seconds fly by before you're both in your birthday suits, you're missing a prime opportunity to extend foreplay and weave in some heavy petting. So next time, adhere to this rule of thumb: Whenever you remove an article of clothing, caress that part of his body at the same time. As you leisurely undo each button on his shirt, pause to stroke the skin you've exposed. As you peel off each sleeve, one at a time, kiss his shoulders and neck. When you pull off his pants, slowly pet each of his legs in the process. Follow sock removal with a foot massage. By the time he's naked (and that could be awhile), his whole body will be humming—and he'll be happy to follow suit.

221   Set a time limit

Agree to engage in foreplay for a certain amount of time (longer than usual, of course) before moving to intercourse. When you make a game out of teetering on the brink until, say, 9:20 p.m., no one's rushing to the finish line, which gives you plenty of time to rev your motors.

222   Try different textures

Remember, your hands are hardly the only things that could be roaming each other's bodies. Tickle him with your hair, letting your locks brush alongside his torso (it'll feel even more amazing down below, so keep going). Or, rather than stripping down

> > Inside the male mind

"One Saturday morning, my wife and I started fooling around, but before it could get hot and heavy, she jumped in the shower. Then we went shopping. But whenever we had a semi-private moment, she'd touch me. By lunchtime all I had on my mind was sex. When we finally got home, we went at it as if we hadn't seen each other in weeks."

—Tim, 35

to your birthday suits, feel each other up *over* your clothing—silk, cotton, cashmere, it's all good (even better if you're not wearing a bra). If you're feeling especially frisky one night, survey the house for anything that might provide some novel sensations—smooth spoons, waxy candles, feathery feather dusters, whatever catches your fancy.

223 Play a game of Keep Away

Use a bathrobe sash to "draw" a line dividing the bed in half. Get as frisky as humanly possible without crossing onto the other side. This will force you to stick to hands-only techniques—at least, for as long as you can bear.

224 Train your sense of touch

In the same way that becoming a food critic requires sharpening your taste buds to tune into the subtle nuances in flavor, becoming a sexual connoisseur takes some sensual schooling. For your first homework assignment, break out the blindfolds. It's a scientific fact: Rob yourself of one source of sensory input, and the others are automatically heightened, which should help you hone in on exactly what feels sensational versus just so-so. Or play the Alphabet Game, where you take turns spelling out words on each other's back or stomach, and then having the recipient guess what you wrote—and which letters rev your engine.

225 Critique each other—constructively

Just as important as knowing what you both like is knowing what you *don't*. To get your point across but soften the blow, try sandwiching each negative between two positives. For example: "You know, I like it when you give attention to my nipples. But sometimes you're too rough. I really love when you massage them softly with your fingers." Take turns giving each other suggestions and listening without interrupting; go back and forth as many times as necessary to get everything off your chest. By the end, you'll never need to put up with nonproductive petting techniques again!

226 Give him a hands-on tutorial

Put your hands over his and glide his mitts over all areas of your body that you want him to touch. Or, put *his* hands over yours and repeat. Either way, he'll be getting some invaluable hands-on advice. They say actions speak louder than words—in this case, they're giving him an encyclopedic amount of info about where, and how, to turn you on.

227 Learn the art of the tease

Once you've identified his hot spots—and he yours—that's when you can *really* start having some fun. Think of teasing as foreplay's evil twin: You caress each other as usual, only do so close, but not quite on, the bull's-eye. Rather than going

SURPRISING SEX FACT!

55 percent of couples kiss and make out on occasion without taking it further, according to a REDBOOK poll.

straight for his nipple, for example, kiss your way around the perimeter, slowly spiraling inward. The nerve endings you ignore (dead center, of course) will become 10 times more sensitive in anticipation.

228 Treat him to all-day foreplay

It's a fact: The longer you engage in foreplay, the more climactic it'll be once you finally culminate the fun. Given that's the case, why not plant the seed at the crack of dawn and let the anticipation grow from there? The minute you wake up next to him, let your hands wander for awhile before you "realize" how late it is and jump out of bed. Then, throughout the day, find excuses to lightly brush against him. Caress his back, chest, or some other favorite body part while sharing household chores or passing each other in the hallway. Let these little tastes of sex percolate, and by nighttime, you'll both be so wound up you'll spring on each other like crazy people.

229 Declare an "everything but" weekend

Take sex out of the equation, and you're bound to get *very* creative turning each other on in other ways. Brace yourself for some wildly imaginative foreplay for a full 48 hours—followed by a sizzling Monday-morning finale.

SURPRISING SEX FACT!

Men—yes, men—crave more foreplay, according to a study from the University of New Brunswick, Canada. In the study, women assumed their partner wanted 13 minutes tops, while lo and behold, men claimed that 18 minutes was ideal.

CHAPTER 12

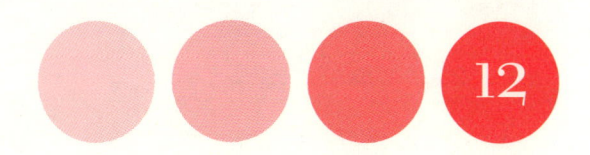

Your head-to-toe guide to erogenous zones

When you and your guy get frisky, it makes sense you'd reach for, well, some pretty obvious body parts. These tried-and-true areas of your anatomy, however, are hardly the only spots that'll get you both hot under the collar. Curious what you're missing? Try taking a detour to some of these more surprising destinations below, and follow a few of our pointers on how to kiss, caress, or (yes) tickle them. While our advice below focuses on how you can do these moves on *him*, most of these techniques can work equally well on either of you, so he should return the favor. Granted, they may not hit home runs for everyone, but still, they're fun for a visit—and if you keep exploring, maybe you'll stumble across some of your *own* moan-worthy zones that deserve to become permanent plays. Have fun!

> ### *Moves men love*
>
> "Molly speaks softly into my ear, saying nice things like, 'You look sexy in that shirt' or 'I love you.' Then she flicks the inside of my ear with the tip of her tongue and takes my earlobe gently between her teeth. That sends shivers down my spine every time."
>
> —Kevin, 34

230 Scalp

While he (or you) is lying down, run your hands through his hair until you're cradling the back of his head. Then feel around gently until you find two slight hollows where his skull meets his neck. These are actually acupressure points, according to Chinese medicine—and, if pressed just so, can fire things up down below. To do that, place two fingers in each of these spots, then lift his head slightly so the weight presses down on your fingertips. This will increase energy flow to the genitals, which may be felt as a warmth or tingling in that area (and you haven't even laid a hand there yet!).

231 Ears

No doubt about it, ear-nibbling is an art form, and this move is its Mona Lisa: First, suck and nibble on his lobe to get him accustomed to the sensation. Then, slowly run your tongue around the outside rim of his ear, following the curve to the indentation at the top. Next, sweep the tip of your tongue around and under the rim, heading back down toward the lobe. Make circles around the inner part of his ear, occasionally blowing warm breaths softly across the wet surface. When he starts squirming with anticipation, point your tongue and slide it in and out of his ear cavity. Done right, it'll elicit goose bumps and the many, many moans of delight.

232 Third eye

According to Eastern religions, this invisible peeper lies smack between his eyebrows and, when "opened," can bring on all sorts of arousing visions. To open it, gently press on the area for 60 seconds. Then ask him what he sees (and don't be surprised if it's something steamy).

233 Nose

Playfully nibble on the tip of his schnoz with your teeth. Here's why he'll like it: Next to your kisser, your sniffer contains more nerve endings than any other part of your face, so it'll enjoy any attention it gets. Plus—here's an interesting bit of trivia for you—your schnoz contains erectile tissue that expands when aroused, further increasing circulation and sensitivity. (Don't worry; this effect occurs mainly *inside* the nasal passages.)

> **SURPRISING SEX FACT!**
>
> Strange, but true: Experts say that stimulating the nose can lead to an endearing affliction called "honeymoon sinusitis," where canoodling couples come down with a puzzling case of nasal congestion.

234   N-spot

Here's an erogenous zone we'll bet neither of you have ever heard of (or felt, for that matter). Kiss, lick, or nibble the crease between his chin and his Adam's apple. When stimulated, this extrasensitive area will activate the nerve endings in his nether regions. He'll never know what hit him!

235   Nape of the neck

The nape of the neck is loaded with nerve endings and carries a symbolic importance as well. In some primitive cultures, they put marks at the nape of the neck to seal in energy. You, however, want to unlock it, and here's how: Place your mouth just inches from the area and breathe a gust of warm air—the tiny hairs there will pick up the motion and give him chills from head to toe.

SURPRISING SEX FACT!

Maybe you've noticed: Feet are insanely ticklish. And while a light touch on these extremities will usually leave the victim screaming for mercy, try it once he's somewhat aroused, and the sensation may actually feel pleasurable.

236 Shoulders

The Shoulder Well, an acupressure point between the tendons on either side of the base of the neck, can store a ton of libido-freezing tension. Knead this area with your thumbs, though, and he'll become putty in your hands.

237 Breastbone

Feel around for an indentation in the breastbone right above the heart. This acupressure point is called the Sea of Tranquility, and for good reason: It can trigger an amazingly relaxed (and romantic) state of mind. Press on it with your fingers and watch him melt.

238 Arms

These limbs possess not just one but *two* major hot spots: the armpit and the inside of the elbow. (In general, all creases on the body are erogenous zones; that includes the back of the knees, the butt crack, where the thighs meet the pelvis, and where the ears meet the skull.) But back to the arms: Since these supersensitive areas can often be ticklish if touched too intensely, stick to feather-light caresses for sublime effects.

239 Chest

A caress of the chest is a classic turn-on tactic—and this massage will *really* make those pecs happy. Sit and have him lie down, placing his head in your lap. Then, slowly slide your hands down his pectoral muscles (the ones right below the clavicle), fanning

> ### SURPRISING SEX FACT!
> Believe it or not, your navel and your clitoris have a surprising amount in common. During the embryonic stage of development, these two regions grew from the same tissue, which means they're neurologically linked in adulthood. In fact, if you stick your finger in your belly button, you may be able to feel a jolt down below.

out toward his armpits. Repeat to his heart's content. (Note: Just because you've got boobs doesn't mean this won't feel wonderful on you as well.)

240 Nipples

Of course, your *own* nipples probably see plenty of action already. But his contain just as many nerve endings as yours—which means you'll *both* love getting some attention here, and the options are endless. Try a gentle pinch, a playful tug, or stroking the area lightly with your fingernails or the palm of your hand. While some men might shy away from having them stimulated because they consider it unmasculine, those who overcome this taboo will be very glad they did. Why not help him out?

241   Navel

Admit it: Belly buttons are so cute they just seem to beg for a little attention. Use your tongue or fingers to delve into this indentation, or if that's too much, kiss or caress your way two to three inches southward. By doing so, you'll hit three reflexology points called the Sea of Energy, which will not only get his erotic engine humming but are linked to fertility.

242   Sacrum

Sure, your tailbone might not *seem* like a sexy area, but these tiny vertebrae right above your buttocks contain the sacral nerve, which shoots straight to your genitals. To trigger a pleasurable chain reaction, have him lie on his stomach as you straddle his thighs. Then, press on the sacrum with your palm or give it a gentle karate-chop-style massage. This will stimulate the sacral nerve and build heat right where it counts.

Moves men love

"I love the way Jaime kisses my hand. First, she holds it, caressing the back of it with her thumb. Next, she raises my hand to her lips and presses them against the back of my hand, and then against my palm. And then she puts her mouth against the inside of my wrist as though she were taking my pulse with her lips. And she always gets that pulse rate up higher."

—Josh, 29

243 Palm of the hand

Crazy-for-each-other couples are joined at the hand as well as the hip: According to the science of reflexology, the center of the palm (right below the middle finger) lies on the pericardium meridian, an energy pathway that's connected to the heart. The upshot? Stimulating the palm will trigger feelings of love and affection. To make your honey's heart go pitter-pat, lightly trace circles counterclockwise over the palm's center. According to Tantric practices, the counterclockwise direction is also counterintuitive, and thereby will produce a fresh, unexpected sensation that will be especially effective.

244 Thighs

Want to get his mojo rising long before you hit X-rated territory? Head for his inner thigh. Starting right above his knee, plant a light-as-a-feather kiss there, then work your way up, increasing the pressure of your lips on his skin the farther you go. Or lean into the thick tendons where his legs join his groin. Either way, you'll get the sexual energy flowing.

SURPRISING SEX FACT!

Electric stimulation of the sacral nerve will trigger an orgasm in 91 percent of women, according to a study by Stuart Meloy, an anesthesiologist in Winston-Salem, North Carolina, who stumbled across this discovery while implanting electrodes there to treat back pain in a patient (who joked afterwards, "You're going to have to teach my husband how to do that!").

SURPRISING SEX FACT!

Ever noticed how your toes twitch reflexively when you hit a high note (thus the term "toe-curling orgasm")? That's because there's a direct neurological link between your privates and your little piggies—especially the biggie. What's more, you can work this reflex in the *other* direction. In other words, stimulating the big toe can actually trigger an orgasm in some lucky people!

245 Soles of the feet

There's a reason why foot rubs feel phenomenal: The bottom of the foot is jam-packed with nerve endings and acupressure points that, after being walked on all day, would love a little TLC. The very best spot to hit for your purposes lies one-third of the way down under the third toe. This spot has been nicknamed the Bubbling Spring; press down here and you may see why: It'll cause energy to "bubble up" the legs and bring his libido to a boil, and fast.

246 Big toe

Since the whole sucking-on-the-big-toe trick is so old hat, we thought we'd fill you in a far fresher (and more effective) maneuver: Gently pinch the sides of his big toe and roll it between your fingers. According to the Chinese practice of reflexology, there are two meridians, or energy pathways, on each side of the big toe that lead upward through the genitals all the way to the pituitary gland. Stimulating these meridians will unblock energy flow and perk up every organ along their paths (for example, your pituitary will start producing more libido-boosting hormones like testosterone, thereby revving your sex drive).

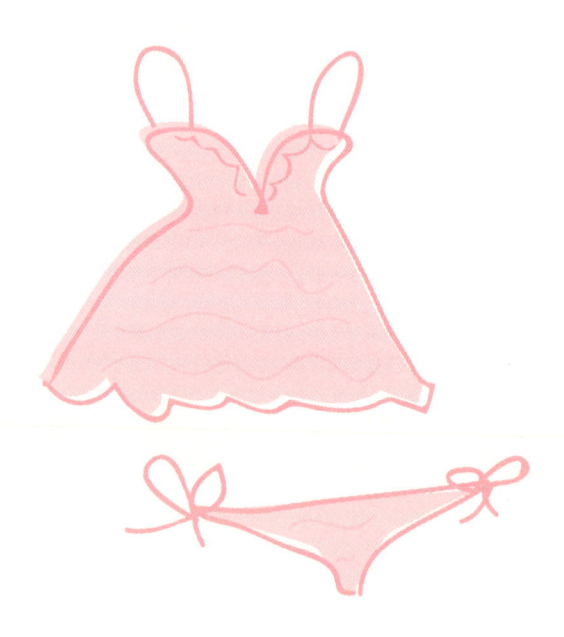

CHAPTER 13

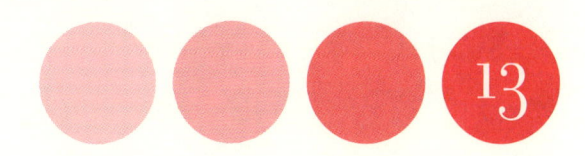

Give him a hand!

Ask yourself: When's the last time you rolled up your sleeves and gave an amazing, so-good-his-eyes-were-in-the-back-of-his-head hand job? If your answer is "high school," "never," or "why bother with hand jobs when there are so many other fun things we could be doing?" we're about to change that. After all, your hands are pretty nimble little instruments. If they can be trained to type over 100 words per minute or play piano concertos, then it stands to reason they can accomplish a lot more on his instrument than your usual up-and-down hand pump, right? Allow us to open your eyes to all the wonderful ways your mitts can work their magic. By the end of this chapter, you'll be all too willing to give the humble hand job the props it truly deserves—and *he'll* be raring to return the favor by flipping to the next chapter.

But first, some hand-job basics to keep in mind...

247 Use lube

May we be blunt? If you're going to polish his apple, saliva will get you only so far. Lubrication is a must to smooth the way. Here, the pros and cons of your options:

Oil-based lubes. Vaseline, hand moisturizer, massage oil, or even olive oil are all handy household options, but be warned: They should *not* be used on you internally or if you might end up having intercourse. Oil in the vagina can linger and cause infections; it can also break down the latex in condoms and diaphragms.

Water-based lubes. Chances are you're already well acquainted with one kind—K-Y Jelly, which most gynos use during pelvic exams. While K-Y has been around forever and can be found at most drug stores, there are plenty of other brands like Astroglide, Liquid Silk, and Slippery Stuff, that are available at drugstores or sex-toy stores and online.

Silicone-based lubes. Long used on lubricated condoms, silicone is now available by the bottle—and good thing, too. Unlike water-based lubes, silicone lasts for hours and doesn't dissolve in water (making it great in the shower or swimming pool). But *don't* use it with silicone sex toys, since it will bind to the toy and get it all gummed up.

PS: Whichever lube you use, keep in mind, it will feel c-c-c-cold if poured directly onto the genitals. So rub it between your hands first to give it a chance to warm up.

248   Rub him right

Handling his joystick just right requires a fine balance of pace and pressure, so keep this rule of thumb in mind: The firmer your grip, the slower your stroke. The lighter your grip, the faster you can go. This will ensure you won't over- or under-stimulate his nerves.

249   Play Show-and-Tell

Want to *really* have a grasp on how he likes his hand jobs delivered? Ask him to toss one off while you watch. If your guy's on the shy side, try this alternative: Place *your* hand on his cash and prizes and ask him to put *his* hand on top of yours and move/squeeze/tug to his heart's content.

SURPRISING SEX FACT!

31 percent of women have a pet name for their partner's penis, according to a REDBOOK poll.

250 Know all his hot spots

We know, we know, his penis *is* one big hot spot. But within that, there are a host of mini moan-worthy zones worth hitting. Here's a rundown:

Glans. Otherwise known as the head of the penis, the glans contains many more nerve endings than the shaft, and will appreciate the extra attention.

Coronal ridge. The edge where the glans meets the shaft is especially sensitive, particularly the spot known as . . .

Frenulum. Located in the center of the underside of the coronal ridge, this little notch is the be-all and end-all of pleasure for many men.

Raphe. On the underside of the shaft is a midline seam that's a zipper of zing-worthy nerve endings.

Scrotum. A.k.a. the family jewels. Handle with care and the results will be pleasurable, not painful.

Seminal vesicles. They'll feel like twigs branching away from the scrotal sack.

Male G-spot. Yup, men have a G-spot too, located at a dime-size area between their scrotum and anus. Press here, and he'll be in heaven.

Anus. This is a no-go zone on many men and for many women. But for those who feel like exploring, we'll show you the ropes below.

Now, the moves that'll rock his world...

251 The Twister

This technique's just your basic hand job, but with a twist—literally—that'll knock his socks off. Wrap your hand around his penis and proceed with your usual up-and-down motion. Only on the upswing as you reach the head, rotate your wrist, then rotate it again on your trip back down. This simple move lavishes attention right where he'll love it most—and since many men might be new to the sensation, don't be surprised if he responds with "Whoa, what was *that*?!" and plenty of puppy-dog gratitude.

SURPRISING SEX FACT!

Ever wonder how often men give themselves a hand? According to a REDBOOK survey, 34 percent of men say they masturbate a few times a month, 31 percent a few times a week, 23 percent almost daily, and 12 percent say never.

One woman's sex secret—revealed

"Unless it's abnormally tiny or abnormally large, size doesn't matter as long as it's used well. If he's aware of positions that allow for maximum stimulation, an 'average' guy can be amazing."

—Candice, 25

252 The Double Fister

Why use one hand when you can use two? Interlace your fingers, then wrap both hands around his penis and move them up and down to deliver double the stimulation that's sure to make him one happy man.

253 Hand-Job Deluxe

There are hand jobs . . . and then there are *hand jobs*. If you want to treat him to the latter one night, try this technique, which hits not just one but a ton of his hot spots (for a full rundown of where those are, see tip #250, "Know all his hot spots," earlier in this chapter). To start, stroke the underside of his penis from base to tip for a few minutes, gliding your fingers along the raphe (the seam of nerves on the underside). Once he's standing at attention (trust us, it won't take long), let your fingers sweep around the coronal ridge, paying special attention to the extrasensitive frenulum on the underside. After a few rounds, return back down the raphe, then repeat. Meanwhile, with your other hand, gently cup and stroke his scrotal sac and seminal vesicles. Since you're targeting his most sensitive spots—and so many at once—even the lightest caress should send him into sensory overload.

254 Circle of Delight

Sometimes focusing all your energy on just one of his sweet spots can be just as arousing (and will convince him you're the most gifted gal he's ever met). So, one night when you want to prove you *really* know what you're doing, gently grab his shaft with your knuckles facing his stomach and, using your thumbs, massage small circles on the frenulum—the area just below the head on the underside of the penis. Since this spot is so sensitive, this move is simple yet *very* effective.

255 Penis Shiatsu

For a completely new sensation, skip stroking and try squeezing. With your thumb and forefinger, form a ring at the base of his penis then tighten the ring for one second. Then release, and move an inch up the shaft and repeat on up to the tip. According

One woman's sex secret—revealed

"I call his Heavy D and the Boys."

—Ana, 30

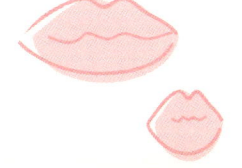

to the Japanese science of shiatsu, the penis contains numerous acupressure points along the shaft that, when pressed, can unlock energy flow and boost circulation (and those are good things as far as erections are concerned).

256 The Web Weaver

Here's one area of your hand we'll bet you've never thought about using down below: the webbing between your fingers. To make the most of it, extend your thumb and forefinger so they form a V and place the shaft of his penis in the crook. Then, move your hand up and down so that the webbing between your fingers gently grazes the shaft. This delicate sensation will feel sublime, and can even resemble how *you* feel south of the border.

257 The Fire Starter

Just when he swears he's seen and felt it all, place your hands on the sides of his penis so they're flat and parallel to each other. Then, gently and lightly move your hands as if you were trying to start a fire with a stick (if you never learned this in Girl Scouts, it's where you quickly rub your hands in opposing directions). By doing this, you'll stimulate his nerve endings in an entirely new way—sideways verses up-and-down—and can create a lot of feel-good friction. (Note: Lots of lube is a must for this move; for suggestions on which types to try, see tip #247, "Use lube," at the start of this chapter.)

258 Play Ball

Many women steer clear of the family jewels, figuring that their efforts here will be painful rather than pleasurable. Not so. Done right, a caress here can feel incredible, provided you take a few precautions. First, encircle the base with thumb and index finger so that the skin on the scrotal sac is taut. Then, lightly caress this area with your fingertips or even your fingernails. If you feel his scrotum contract toward his body, congratulations! That means he's enjoying it.

259 The Male G-Spot Jump-start

Most men don't even know they *have* a G-spot, much less where it is. Now, how thankful do you think he'll be if you found it for him? To activate, ask your guy to lie down and prop his feet on your shoulders as you kneel between his legs. Run your hand along the muscular band of flesh between his scrotum and his anus, searching for a slightly indentation or dimple. Bingo! Press on this area to send him skyward.

SURPRISING SEX FACT!

Does the size of a man's member really matter? Men will be relieved to know that the majority of women (56 percent) in a REDBOOK poll say no.

260 The Backdoor Bonanza

Okay, first things first: If your guy wants to be penetrated anally, that does *not* mean he's gay. Now that that's out of the way, let's get to the good stuff: The reason men may find this enjoyable is because it stimulates his prostate gland, a super-sensitive spot located two inches in on the front wall of the anal cavity. If you're open to exploring this taboo territory, make sure to ask first if he feels the same way (this is *not* the kind of thing you want to spring on him as a surprise). If he's game, you may need to invest in a few accessories: Lube for sure (without it, ouch) and, if you like, latex finger cots from the drugstore or condoms to place over your fingers, which help prevent internal skin tears and offer you a little extra covering, too. On the big night, make sure to butter him up first with tons of foreplay . . . then proceed *slooowly*, tracing circles around the perimeter. Once you're in, pause for a moment so he can get used to the sensation, then try stroking or pressing on the prostate and see how he reacts (which will most likely be with pinwheel-eyed enthusiasm).

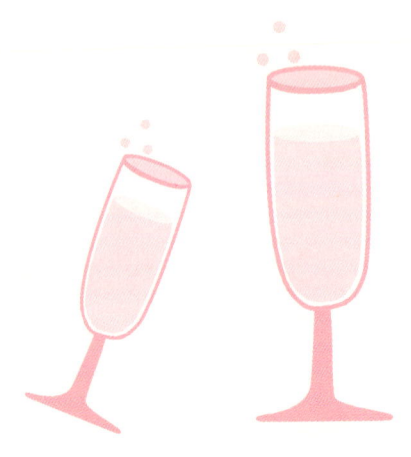

CHAPTER 14

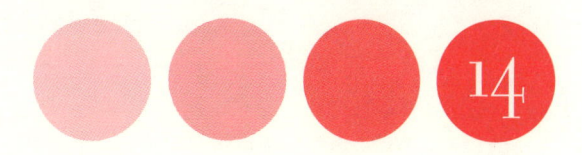

How *he* can give *you* a hand

In the previous chapter, we slipped you some tricks on how to give him the happiest of happy endings, and chances are, he's dying to demonstrate he's got a few tricks up his sleeve, too. Well, why not help him out by passing along a few of these pointers? Most men will be astounded to learn there are tons of techniques to try beyond your basic below-the-belt finger wiggle. Heck, *you'll* be astounded—you don't know what you've been missing until you've felt a few of these moves. Fasten your seatbelts and have fun!

But first, some basics rules to keep in mind . . .

261 We can't say it enough: Use lube

Lube may be important for him, but it's also critical for you. Let's face it, we all have days when our own resources run a little, well, dry—and not necessarily because we aren't turned on. Women's natural lubrication levels ebb and flow based on their menstrual cycle, medication they're taking (anti-histamines will dry you out), whether they've been drinking or smoking, and other factors. Saliva may work in a pinch, but it evaporates quickly, leaving you back where you started. So, to avoid a rub-down that feels more like rug burn, keep a tube of lube handy (for suggestions on which types to try, turn to tip #247, "Use lube," at the start of the previous chapter).

262 Watch the nails

Scrrrrape. Not exactly what you want happening when he's petting your petunia. To figure out if his fingernails are so long or jagged they'll do more damage than good down there, have him curve his fingers and rub his gums above his top teeth. If he can feel his nails, you will, too, and it's time for a trim.

263 Show him how it's done

That's right, masturbate in front of your man. Not only will he love the sight of you being so unabashedly indulgent, it will teach him a *ton* about what he should be doing to you down below. If the mere thought of doing this makes you blush in embarrassment, there is an alternative: Put his hands on your privates, place your mitts on top of his, and move them the way you'd like.

264 Explore all your hot spots

Even the most savvy guy can feel a little lost south of the border—what's more, many women aren't even aware of all the destinations worth visiting. To help you both out, here's a travel itinerary:

Mons pubis. This furry mound just north of your main attractions may not seem worth mentioning, but it serves an important function. Like a shock absorber, it keeps the highly sensitive areas below from receiving too much stimulation during intercourse. Plus, if jiggled just so, this area can also bring on a Big O. More on that later.

Clitoral head. Hands down, this little nub is the center of a woman's sexual universe. Packed with 8,000 nerve endings (twice as many as in the head of the penis), it's actually so sensitive that, prior to orgasm, it seeks refuge from all the hubbub and retracts under the next point of interest on our tour.

Clitoral hood. A fold of skin that covers the clitoral head and offers added protection for this touchy territory. However, like a convertible car hood, it can be pulled back in case your clitoris feels up for a more intense ride.

Labia majora. The outer folds of skin surrounding the vagina, usually covered with pubic hair. Sure they're sensitive, but they're stalwart as WWF wrestlers compared to their neighbors.

Labia minora. These smooth folds of skin inside the labia majora are so responsive that once roused they swell in size and change color from pink to purple.

G-spot. This quarter-sized area located a couple inches in on the front wall of the vagina has been a hotbed of controversy since its discovery in 1944. Does it really exist? Can it really induce earthshaking orgasms that make women, um, ejaculate? Well, it's certainly worth a visit to see for yourself.

Perineum. Located beneath the vagina and above the anus, this spot is also quaintly known as the "taint" since "taint one nor the other"—but 'tis worth a visit.

Anus. Maybe yours is closed for business, but if not, we've got some ideas for you.

SURPRISING SEX FACT!

What's more of a turn-on: giving or receiving oral sex? According to a REDBOOK poll, 39 percent of women say they prefer to give, with 61 percent saying they would rather receive.

Now, the moves that'll rock your world . . .

265 Rock around the Clock

This move is the perfect warm-up, where he uses his index finger to trace tiny circles around your clitoris, stopping at 12, 3, 6, and 9 o'clock. Strange, but true: Many women seem to like the 2- or 3-o'clock positions the best.

266 Pitcher's Mound

For women who find direct stimulation to their clitoris or vagina too overwhelming, this technique is the perfect alternative. Get your guy to rest his whole hand on your mons pubis (right where your pubic hair is) and move the *entire* area in slow circles. By doing so, he indirectly stimulates the clitoris and gets your engine purring without going overboard.

267 Stick-'Em-Up

Have him insert his index (and perhaps middle) finger into your vagina but keep his thumb cocked like a gun. That way, it will hit your clitoris every time he delves deep, which should get you locked and loaded in no time.

268 Dial-an-Orgasm

Warning: This technique requires a *very* soft touch, but done right, it's your hotline to heaven. To start, have him press his hand onto your mons pubis and pull up. This should cause the clitoral hood and surrounding tissue to retract, revealing your clitoris front and center. Then, using an index finger and thumb, he gently pinches the sides of your clitoris then rotates his fingers as if he were adjusting a dial. Stay tuned for some *very* intense sensations.

269 Tap Dance

If you're on the brink of a Big O and want to linger in this delicious limbo, light tapping on the clitoral hood with one or two fingers may be the ticket. These little love pats are brief but invigorating enough to keep you happy—and if he taps fast enough, he may tip you over the edge.

270 Lip Service

Your inner labia rarely get much hands-on attention, but you're about to change that. Have him gently pinch them together, pull them away from your body so the skin is taut, then wiggle them from side to side. Not only will this get your blood pumping southward, but since the inner labia are attached to the clitoral hood, he'll be indirectly stimulating your love button above.

271 The G-spot Grazer

A quick history lesson: Back in 1944, Dr. Ernst Grafenberg "discovered" a spot in the vagina that, rumor had it, could produce earthshaking, angels-singing orgasms and even cause women to ejaculate. Maybe you'll agree, maybe you won't—the spot's sensitivity levels vary from individual to individual—but here's how you can find out where you fall on this spectrum. Have your guy insert a finger into your vagina and feel on the front wall for a rough, quarter-sized patch about two inches in. Then, have him wiggle his finger in a "come here" motion. This may prompt a need to pee; if so, go to the bathroom then try again. It may *still* prompt a need to pee, but ride through this sensation and pretty soon, you may start feeling *really* good. And if your orgasm *does* erupt in a literal shower of gratitude, don't worry, this milky discharge is not urine, but comes from the paraurethral glands. Most guys, if warned beforehand it might happen, will find it totally cool (and if he doesn't, please be sure to point out how often *he's* prompted a sheet cleaning).

272 Give Me a C

As the name suggests, he forms a C with his hand, inserting his thumb into your vagina while his fingers curve up and rest on your clitoris. Then, he rocks his hand from side to side, stimulating your G-spot *and* C-spot at once.

> **SURPRISING SEX FACT!**
>
> 68 percent of women say they've found their G-spot, says a REDBOOK survey.

273 The Perineum Pinch

With palm facing down, he inserts an index finger into your vagina and presses down, then uses his thumb to press up on your perineum, the area right below your vagina. By doing this, he's in effect stimulating the perineum from *both* sides, inside and out—and that will make you very, very happy.

274 The Backdoor Boogie

We'll bet many of you are wincing and flipping the page at this point, but whether you've had an unsavory experience in your past or never bothered because you just *know* you're not into it, set your judgments aside for a sec and hear us out. Done right— we repeat, done *right*—anal penetration can be very pleasurable. Unlike men, we don't have a supersensitive prostate gland back there to pay a visit, but still, *all* body orifices are packed with nerve endings that appreciate a little attention. So if you're at all curious, go ahead, give it a try, making sure to take these precautions: (1) use lube, (2) go slow, and (3) keep in mind, anything that's been in your exit should not subsequently go in your vagina, since this can cause an infection. To ward off that possibility, he should wash his hands before you get busy and use one hand exclusively for back road excursions, reserving his other hand for the front. Or he can place latex finger cots or condoms over his fingers, then take them off once he moves on to other areas of your anatomy.

CHAPTER 2

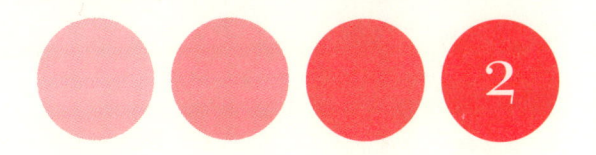

Blow him away!

Don't get us wrong: Men love *all* oral sex. If you're down there, he's in heaven, period. Still, don't you want to blow past his expectations and introduce him to levels of bliss far beyond what he dared to dream could exist? Totally doable—just take a tip or two from this chapter, which will get you using your tongue, lips, and, yes, even teeth on his prime real estate in ways you've never imagined (nor has he, which is *really* saying something). Ladies, prepare to plaster a perma-grin on his face and yours.

But first, some basic rules to keep in mind . . .

275 Maintain a little eye contact

Believe it or not, men *can* get a little lonely up there. So, make sure to glance up and hold his gaze every once in awhile. Add a devilish gleam in your eye, and he'll be in heaven.

276 Lend a helping hand

Let's face it, your mouth can only cover so much ground (the average penis is five to six inches, while the average mouth is only two to three inches—you do the math). That's why the very best oral sex usually incorporates some hands-on action to pick up the slack. So, feel free to mix-and-match the moves in this chapter with those in chapter 11. Or make an O with your hand, place it on your lips, and move them in tandem. This will create the illusion that you're taking him *all* in while in reality it's more like three-fifths. Pretty good trick, huh?

277 Know the science of suction

Ever wonder why they're called blow jobs when you're actually doing the exact opposite—sucking? Anyway, for anyone who can't quite figure out how to do it, suction is created by placing the back of your tongue on the roof of your mouth then sliding it backward to create a vacuum. Now, we all know suction's a crucial ingredient to oral sex, but keep in mind, we can only really suck on the first inch and a half. Take in any more, and your tongue must drop to accommodate it, nullifying those

Hoover-esque effects. Don't worry, though—many men find too much suction a turnoff. To find out how much he likes, ask him to suck on your fingers with the intensity he'd like you to use down yonder. Then fine-tune your technique accordingly.

278 Prep the area so it's palatable

Granted, there are plenty of reasons to *not* like giving oral sex. That doesn't mean you just have to sit there and suffer, since there are plenty of ways to circumvent these unsavory aspects. For example, pounce *right after* he's taken a shower. Ask him to trim his pubic hair, or offer to do it yourself. If you're worried about your gag reflex, you can prevent this by making sure *you're* in control of the motion, not him. And if swallowing isn't up your alley, have him stage his release on your chest, which is nice eye candy for him and won't muck up your hair.

SURPRISING SEX FACT!

Eating melon, kiwi, pineapple, strawberries, or even celery will give men's semen a sweeter taste; alcohol and cigarettes will make it more bitter. And if you're worried it's fattening, don't be—on average, one ejaculation contains only 6 calories.

Now, the moves that'll rock his world...

279 The Backstroke

Chances are, you're already using your tongue in all sorts of tantalizing ways down below. But here's one thing you probably haven't considered: using the *underside* of your tongue instead. Its soft, silky texture will feel especially sublime on the frenulum—a super-sensitive spot located below the head of his penis in the center of the underside of the coronal ridge, (for more precise directions to this erogenous zone and others, turn to tip #250, "Know *all* his hot spots"). Here's what to do: Holding the base of his penis and resting your chin on the underside of his shaft for stability, place the underside of your tongue on this sweet spot and quickly swipe it from side to side like a windshield wiper. Precise as surgery and yet very potent, this move is a great way to kick things off.

280 The Ice-Cream Cone Technique

We think you can imagine what this looks like. Make your tongue as flat as possible (it'll cover more territory that way), then slowly run it along his pride and joy from base to tip. Take your time, leave no spot unlicked, and this move will look as delightful as it feels.

281 The Rhythm Method

Once you're down there and going at it, pacing becomes important, and this move will show him you've got that base covered. Rather than just bobbing up and down at a constant speed, start with five slow bobs, then move to four slow bobs and one fast, then three slow and two fast, and so on. Once you've reached five fast ones, revert back to five slow, then repeat. This move adds variation but also builds anticipation—two of the most basic components to great oral sex.

282 Wind in the Willows

To wake up his nerve endings in an entirely new way, take a break from your usual warm-and-wet routine, pucker your lips, and blow. Shivers of bliss should ensue.

283 The Pearly Gates

As a general rule, teeth and penises don't play well together, but this technique (and the next one, for that matter) is one very sexy exception. Lick your front teeth, tilt your head sideways, then press the flat of your chompers against the shaft, running them up and down its length. Sound sketchy? Truth is, as long as you avoid sharp, pointed edges that can scrape the skin, he'll appreciate *any* new textures you try on him. And believe it or not, this move will actually feel smooth (they don't call your teeth pearly whites for nothing).

284 The Tug of Love

Nibble your way up the side of his penis as if it were corn on the cob, taking the skin lightly between your lips or teeth and tugging gently. Believe it or not, it is possible to pinch the skin here without inducing pain: Done right, these little love nips will galvanize his nerve endings—and make you look like a bit of an animal (trust us, that's a good thing).

285 Oral Sex on the Rocks

Put an ice cube in your mouth before diving down. The heat of your mouth combined with the occasional flashes of chilliness will keep him on his toes.

286 The Mint-in-Mouth Trick

Rumors abound that popping a few Altoids prefellatio can result in a "curiously strong" send-off. But is it true? Well, science seems to support this claim: The menthol that causes the pleasant tingling in your mouth should work on *all* mucous membranes, which include the nostrils and those naughtier bits below. So, go ahead and give it a try—or, to take the sensation to next level, take a swig of club soda along with a mint, which will create a fizzing, bubbly eruption in your mouth that he's bound to enjoy. (And no, it's not dangerous.)

287 Upside-down Oral Sex

Lie on your back on the bed or a couch and lean your head off the edge. Meanwhile, he stands, inserts his penis into your mouth, then moves it in and out while you remain still. Not only will he enjoy controlling the motion (and you'll learn a ton about what he'd like *you* to do down below), but by leaning back, you create a straight path from your mouth to your throat, making it easier for him to delve deep. Don't worry, we're not talking *Deep Throat* deep. If you're afraid he'll induce your gag reflex, tell him to take it slow and place your hands on his buttocks or pelvis to steer him a little. (Random factoid: When a man controls the action it's actually not called fellatio, but irrumination, but most guys don't really care what it's called; they're too occupied with the fact that it feels *amazing*.)

288 The Big W

Now that you've spent plenty of time on his most prized real estate, let us turn for a moment to a neighboring area that rarely gets as many visitors: the scrotum. Whether you steer clear of his testicles because you're afraid they're too sensitive or just have

One woman's sex secret—revealed

"Even though I love receiving, giving oral sex is the bigger turn-on. I love that look on his face—you know, the eternally grateful one—and the sounds he makes."

—Jillian, 24

no clue what to do with them, this technique will get you touring the highlights without too much effort. Starting with your tongue at the top left-hand corner, trace a path down along the side and, once you reach the bottom, do a U-turn and swoop up the middle seam between his testicles. Then backtrack down the seam, around the bottom, and up the right side. Essentially, you'll be tracing a large W, which, in his mind, can stand for only one thing: "Wow!"

CHAPTER 16

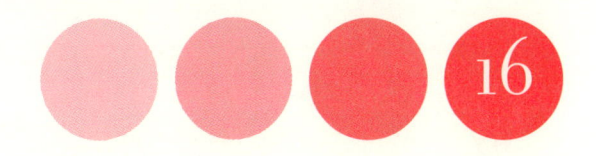

The lowdown on going down

For most women, oral sex is like a free day pass at the spa: It's an opportunity to kick back, relax, and let others do the work. What's more, most men are enthusiastically up for the job and eager to learn what they can do to guarantee you're having a good time. Why not improve the odds that'll happen by slipping him a few pointers? Whether his oral-sex skills could stand a little improvement or are stellar already, the tips in this chapter will give him plenty of bright ideas that are bound to impress you!

First, some basic rules...

289 Let his tongue take breaks

Does his tongue tend to get tired before you trip the light fantastic? Tell him to keep it still and wag his whole head in a "yes" or "no" motion. That way, he can give his tongue a rest without interrupting the fun. Or have him switch to or incorporate some manual maneuvers from chapter 12 to keep things rolling long enough for you to cross the finish line.

290 Trim the hedges

To make yonder valleys inviting to potential visitors, cut or shave your pubic hair or book a waxing appointment at the salon. Not only does this allow him to avoid hair-in-teeth troubles, it also makes your below-the-belt hot spots much easier to access (for a full rundown of the areas he should hit, turn to tip #264, "Explore all your hot spots," near the beginning of chapter 14).

One woman's sex secret—revealed

"I love the way my husband responds when I give oral sex. But when he's the giver—let's just say that he is very, very good!"

—Rachel, 22

291 Experiment with different positions

While women typically receive oral sex lying on their back with legs spread on the bed, that's hardly the only option—and since oral sex is such an intense sensation, it's good to explore alternatives to see what floats your boat. Try it with your legs closer together, or curled up near your head, or hanging off the bed. Since this changes the angle at which your genitals meet his mouth, the very same tongue move may feel remarkably different. Or, if you crave a little more control, hop on top so he's beneath you, which allows you to raise and lower your body depending on how much stimulation you'd like to get.

292 Tune him into your body language

As hard as they try to suss it out, many men are clueless about how much stimulation you need. As a result, they often go overboard (ouch!) or tread so lightly you want to tear your hair out. To get him on target, teach him to take a tip from your hips. If, for example, your hips are shrinking *away* from his mouth or your legs are folding in, that means you're being overstimulated and he should lay off a little. If, on the other hand, your pelvis is arching up to meet his mouth or your legs are widening, that means you want more, more, more! Fill him in on this tidbit of pelvic vocabulary, and suddenly he'll see the light—and everything he does will feel *just right*.

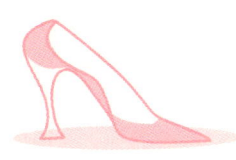

Now, the moves that'll rock your world . . .

293 The Lollipop Lick

For this move, he makes his tongue as wide and flat as possible then takes his sweet time (a few seconds at least) licking you from your perineum (beneath your vulva) up to your clitoris. Not only is this a great way to warm things up, but by covering so much ground and going slow, he can start honing in on your personal hot spots based on where he is when you moan. Tell him to take note.

294 The Soft Pedal

As you've probably noticed, the clitoris is a veritable mine field of sensitivity. All the more reason to try this subtle move: Have him place the *underside* of his tongue on your clitoris and swipe it from side to side. It will feel sublime in comparison to his tongue's rough upper half; and can limber up the area for more vigorous oral acrobatics later.

SURPRISING SEX FACT!

73 percent of men have a pet name for their partner's genitals or breasts, according to a REDBOOK poll.

295 The Wheel of Fortune

Many men, in an effort to add pizzazz to their oral maneuvers, have resorted to writing out the entire alphabet with their tongue. We certainly think that deserves an E for effort, but the truth is, your guy may be wasting his time with a lot of letters that

> ### Inside the male mind
>
> "While giving her oral sex, sometimes I do the ABCs with my tongue and think about what letter I stopped on when she orgasmed."
>
> —Doug, 37

don't do it for you, and short-changing you on those that will send you skyward. So why not find out your favorites, then set them on repeat? According to women, a capital letter F (one stroke up, then two sideways strokes, on the top and bottom of the clitoris) does wonders. So does an H (two up-and-down strokes interspersed with one sideways swipe). Or who knows, maybe you're an O-girl who just loves getting it from all sides. You'll never know until you try—and trust us, it's one writing project he won't mind collaborating on one bit.

296 The Elvis Impersonator

Don't worry, even if your guy's never seen The King in action, he shouldn't have a problem copping this move. In a nutshell, all he has to do is raise his lip in a snarl. Voilà, instant Elvis. Then, he presses his top gums against your clitoris, slowly shaking his head back and forth. Up until now, we'll bet, you've probably never wondered, *Hmm, what would his gums feel like down there?*

But we can vouch for the fact that they actually provide a pretty interesting texture snuggled up on your tender spots. Enough so that Elvis is bound to get an encore.

297 The Suction Cup

While sucking is generally thought of as something women do to men in the oral sex arena, your guy can—and should—try it on you, too. Just have him place his lips around your clitoris and gently draw it in. This will increase blood flow to the area, making your clitoris even more sensitive to all your guy has to offer. (It's about time we girls got our fair share of this technique!)

298 The Pointillist

Remember back in art class when you learned about Pointillism—a genre of painting where images were created from thousands of tiny dots of color? Your guy can create a similar masterpiece on *you* by using the principles behind this technique. Instead of "brushing" against your canvas, have him point his tongue and dot the area—a teasing touch that can be especially effective when you're on the edge of orgasm and want to linger on this delicious precipice.

SURPRISING SEX FACT!

When a REDBOOK poll asked whether it's more fun to give or receive oral sex, the majority of men—55 percent—said they'prefer to give. Meanwhile, only 39 percent of women feel the same way. Looks like men are more generous than we are!

299 Below-the-Belt Liplock

Maybe you think the whole tongue-in-the-vagina thing is a waste of time—especially given he's got plenty of larger options at his disposal. Still, what you might be overlooking is that the vaginal opening is very sensitive, and will enjoy an up-and-down or side-to-side tongue-lashing. Try it and see; or for bonus points, have him suck the inner labia into his mouth while he penetrates with his tongue. The effects, some women claim, are absolutely incredible.

300 The Hot-'n'-Cold Combo

To pull this one off, he'll need props—something cold (like ice water) and something hot (like coffee or tea). He takes a sip of one or the other, then places his hot (or cold) lips on your privates. This will get your neurons firing afresh to an entirely new stimulus—temperature—and alternating from one extreme to the other will only amplify the effects.

301 The Mint-in-Mouth Trick

Thanks to widespread rumors of the Altoid/oral sex connection, tons of women have chomped on menthol candies before going down on their guy. But what you might not know is that the tingling sensation these mints produce works even better on *you*, since menthol can more easily penetrate the mucous membranes of your genitals than his. So, make sure your guy gives you a taste of what those "curiously strong" mints feel like down below.

302   The Hummingbird

The next time he's down on you, encourage him to start humming a little ditty—"Happy Birthday," "It Had To Be You," "I Will Survive," it really doesn't matter. Sure, it may seem weird, but you'll both change your tune once you feel the results. Activating the vocal chords will create a buzz on his lips, turning them into a vibrator. If he can't bring himself to stage this strange performance and would prefer a more natural approach, letting loose a long moan or two will also do the trick.

CHAPTER 17

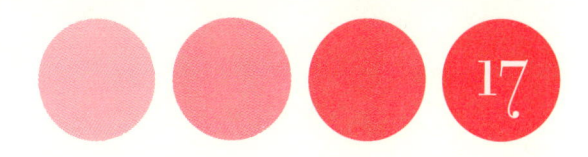

Assume the position! 22 to try

When couples think about experimenting with new sex positions, it's easy to, well, worry a little. Maybe you're wondering, Can I really hoist my leg up there? What if he throws his back out? Is all the potential pain and suffering worth contorting into some pretzelesque pose? Never fear, trying new poses is hardly as difficult or death-defying as it's often cracked up to be. Most times, all it takes is the smallest twists to your favorites to deliver a bigger bang for your buck. As proof, check out these options and try a few that sound like they're up your alley (and have a go at some that don't, too). Plus, for you more flexible, adventurous sorts, we've thrown in plenty of more challenging poses in case you want to give 'em a go. Make sure to stretch beforehand. And good luck!

Enjoy missionary the most? Then try these new twists...

303 The Burning Bridge

Lift your hips so they're off the bed, either keeping your feet planted or wrapping your legs around his waist. The new tilt of your pelvis is bound to expose your most sensitive spots (like your clitoris) much better than the standard missionary.

304 The Lazy Man's Burning Bridge

Stick a pillow under your butt—same new pelvic tilt, same sensitive-spot rubbing, but a lot less work than The Burning Bridge.

305 The Golden Gate

Raise your legs and drape them over his shoulders so your knees or calves are on either side of his head (don't worry, it's not as hard as it sounds). Or bend your knees and place your feet flat against his chest. Thrusting is effortless for him in this position, so prepare for a wild ride!

306 The One-Lane Highway

Once he's inside you, squeeze your legs together so his thighs are straddling yours. The snugger fit will make your vagina feel tighter, his penis feel bigger, and create a whole lot of friction you'll both enjoy.

307 The One-Legged Stork

Raise just one leg so it rests on his torso while keeping the other flat on the bed. This position has two things going for it: easy thrusting, plus now there's room for you (or him) to reach down and manually stimulate your clitoris for added kicks.

308 The Crazy CAT

In truth, the missionary position doesn't always give women enough clitoral contact to reach her peak—but leave it to a sexual researcher (Edward Eichel) to change that by inventing the Coital Alignment Technique (CAT). To do it, have your guy slide his torso up a few inches so he rocks, rather than thrusts, into you, keeping his pubic bone connected to yours at all times. The added clitoral stimulation is scientifically proven to up your enjoyment level.

Moves men love

"Karla has a thing about pillows. We have about a dozen down pillows on our bed, and she uses them for adjusting her position during intercourse. But she also props me up with pillows behind my back when she performs oral sex. That way I can see everything she's doing. Wow!"

—Bruce, 40

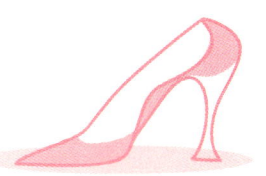

Prefer to hop on top? Then try these new twists...

309 The Amazing Arc

Slide your legs down so they're straddling his thighs rather than his torso. Arch your back so you're nearly perpendicular to the bed. The arc shape of your body will put maximum pressure on your clitoral area, which may send you overboard in no time.

310 The Sumerian Squat

Experts claim this was the signature sex position of the ancient Mesopotamian goddess Inanna, and we have to say, Inanna was onto something. Keeping the soles of your feet on the bed and your knees up, lower yourself onto your husband's penis. Then bend your legs slightly to move up and down. Not only does this give you both a great view of the action below, but this take-charge pose really does make you look like a goddess.

311 The Reverse Cowgirl

In this position, you spin so you're facing his feet, then go at it with your torso perpendicular to the bed (or you can lean back against his chest). This, of course, gives him a great view of your derriere—and the new angle of him inside you can create a whole host of sweet new sensations.

Like it best from behind?
Then try these new twists . . .

312 The Crouching Tiger

Being on all fours while your partner takes you from behind is already erotically animalistic, but you can make it even more sexually charged by lowering your chest to the bed. This angle elongates and tightens your vagina, resulting in an even more snug, more tantalizing fit.

313 The Standing Tiger

Move to the edge of the bed so he's standing rather than kneeling behind you. Or you can *both* stand while you lean on the bed. With feet planted firmly on the ground, as opposed to a cushiony mattress, the thrusting will feel hard, fast, and *extremely* satisfying.

314 The Sleeping Tiger

In this position, you lie on the bed on your stomach; he lies on top of you. Experiment with having both or just one of his legs between yours, or having your legs between his for a variety of sizzling sensations.

Find sideways sex most satisfying? Then try these new twists...

315 The Swinging Bishop

When you're in the spooning position with your back to his, lift your top leg and have him hold it, or drape your leg over his. This allows for even deeper penetration—and gives you both great access to your clitoris if you've craving extra encouragement.

316 X Marks the Spot

Shift your bodies so they form more of an X. Both of your legs should be on top of his hips. You are lying on your back and he is lying on his side. From here, you can keep your legs together and angled up toward the ceiling, or spread them so one's extended toward his head and the other toward his feet, or somewhere in between. This position leaves plenty of room for either of you to reach for your clitoris and give it a rubdown, but with an added benefit: You can open or close your legs to adjust how much stimulation you get. How's that for personalized service?

Girl talk tip-off

"Sideways is the most relaxing, since neither of us has to do much work. Plus, it gives him great access to my breasts and other erogenous zones."

—Dina, 30

SURPRISING SEX FACT!

Which sex position do men dig most? According to a REDBOOK poll, here's a rundown:
38 percent like it best from behind
36 percent hope a woman will hop on top
20 percent prefer missionary
6 percent are suckers for sideways

317 The Kissing Goldfish

You don't have to spoon to make sideways sex work. Believe it or not, it *is* possible to have sex sideways while facing each other—just lift your leg so he can scoot in there. Movement will be limited to grinding rather than thrusting, but these more subtle movements can be highly stimulating, especially since his every hip wiggle will be hitting your clitoris front and center. Plus (attention romance junkies) since you're facing each other, you can kiss and gaze into each other's eyes.

Up for even more of a challenge? Give these sex positions a try...

318 The Wally Wallbanger

Have your guy lift you up and press your back against the wall, or just lean against it, raise one leg, and have him bend his knees so he can enter. Either way, this position carries all the spontaneity and excitement of sex while standing (couldn't even wait long enough to lie down, could you?) but without the precarious balancing issues. Even if he's holding you up, he won't have to carry your full weight.

319 Stairway to Heaven

Stairways are great for sex, and here's why: All you need to do is lift one leg so it's draped over the banister then go at it in the standing position easy as pie. Who knows? Try it out on your way up to the bedroom and you may never make it that far.

320 The Wheelbarrow

This one's not for the weak of limb, but those who can swing it will feel very studly. You kneel on all fours, then your guy lifts your legs on each side of his waist like, well, wheelbarrow handles. Then he plows ahead. If you thought regular old sex from behind wins points for its animalistic flair, this position will *really* wow you.

321 The Yab-Yum

In Tantric tradition, this position—practiced by the gods—is said to lead to spiritual enlightenment (or, at least, to some very soul-stirring orgasms). To do it, sit facing each other, then scoot forward so your privates meet in the middle and your legs are draped over his. Then rock into each other as you gaze into each other's eyes and embrace.

322 The Table Turner

Desk, kitchen counter, dining room table—they're all fair game. Just lie on your back with your butt on the edge while he stands and delivers. Try it with your legs apart, or together propped on his shoulder, or with him holding your ankles for added comfort and control.

SURPRISING SEX FACT!

And which sex position do women prefer?
37 percent enjoy missionary the most
32 percent prefer to hop on top
25 percent like it best from behind
6 percent are most satisfied sideways

323 The Leaning Tower of Pisa

Less delicate folks might call this the Pile Driver, and while we've tried to attach a gentler eponym, this move is definitely not for the faint of heart. Your guy kneels, grabs your legs and hoists them up onto his shoulders, then enters you while you're practically doing a headstand below. A neck ache may ensue over time, but while it lasts, it's definitely impressive and will give the guy an "I'm king of the world!" rush. Meanwhile, you'll get to experience your own rush—of blood to your head, for starters, but also of getting manhandled in the most satisfying way.

324 Upside-down Diamond

Pull this off, and postcoital high-fives are in order. Lie on your back. Placing your hands on your lower back, lift the lower part of your torso so it's reaching for the ceiling. Split your legs so they form a V midair. He stands and straddles that V with one leg on each side before joining genitals. No, it's not very comfortable, but visually it's a stunner and worth it for bragging rights alone.

SURPRISING SEX FACT!

In studies done on the Coital Alignment Technique, an astounding 77 percent of female subjects reached orgasm this way often or always, and 36 percent did so simultaneously with their partners.

CHAPTER 18

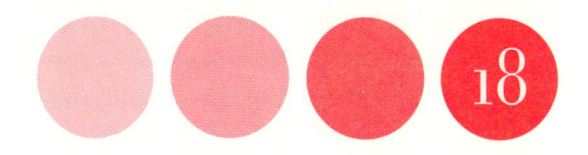

O my! Everything you need to know about orgasms

No doubt about it, orgasms feel *good*. There's a reason you can't spell the words "hot" or "love" or "ohmigodohmigodohohoh . . . " without lots and lots of Os. And yet, most women view their ability (or inability) to reach awe-inspiring peaks as pure luck of the draw. It's as if we think an Orgasm Fairy comes down and blesses some lucky gals with tons of earthquaking Os and the rest of us with a handful of so-so ones—and, worse yet, that there's not a heckuva lot we can do to change our fate. But O contraire! There is something—in fact, there are plenty of things—you can do. Whether you want to make yours bigger, bring 'em on faster, go for multiples, or shoot for a simultaneous O-fest with your one-and-only, the info below is bound to help.

325 Breathe

It's simple: Muscles need oxygen to function properly, and that includes the muscles that contract during orgasm (the pubococcygeal, or PC, muscles, to be exact). And yet, many women, as they approach their peak, do the exact opposite of what would help them out—they pant shallowly or, worse yet, hold their breath (a common impulse if you're trying to concentrate). Instead, take deep breaths through your mouth instead of your nose, then stay tuned for a breathtaking finale.

> **SURPRISING SEX FACT!**
>
> What exactly happens in your body when you orgasm? Well, your pubococcygeal (PC) muscles spasm rhythmically at 0.8 second intervals. Your heart rate accelerates to as fast as 180 beats per minute. And you'll burn as many as 200 calories if it's preceded by a half-hour of lovemaking (if you don't climax, you'll burn roughly half that many calories).

326 Do Kegels during intercourse

No doubt you've heard about Kegel exercises (if not, flip back to tip #111, "The Classic Kegel," in chapter 6), the below-the-belt workout that can strengthen your PC muscles and orgasms along with it. Maybe you even make a point of doing 30 reps while, say, sitting in traffic or walking the dog. Next time, though, consider doing your Kegels *during* intercourse: Contract your PC muscles as he enters and relax them as he withdraws. Given that an orgasm is essentially a series of muscular contractions, this exercise can actually help trigger yours—why wait when you can give it a jump-start?

327 Be pushy

If you've tried flexing your PC muscles during intercourse and loved the results, then try the opposite: Rather than contracting upward, bear down on these muscles to register some new rumblings on your Richter scale. Why? It'll force your G-spot—the extrasensitive area along the front wall of your vagina—closer to your vaginal opening and get it rubbing even more snugly against his equipment. Ever heard guys complain that the G-spot is hard to reach? Well, in essence, you're bringing your G-spot to him. What's not to love?

328 Teach *him* to try Kegels, too

Does your guy tend to reach the Point of No Return way before you—despite doing his darndest to hang in there by thinking about baseball or icebergs? Trust us, there are better tactics to keep him on hold. For one, those Kegel exercises we were just raving about also give *him* control over his own PC muscles, and

SURPRISING SEX FACT!

How do women most easily achieve the Big O? According to a REDBOOK poll, here's a rundown of the most common ways:
29 percent through oral sex
25 percent through intercourse
18 percent through manual stimulation during sex
17 percent through masturbation
11 percent through a vibrator

when he lets loose. Tell him to flex these muscles 30 times daily—like you, he can locate these muscles by stopping the flow of urine. They can also stop the flow of, um, other things. Bye-bye, baseball, hello, marathon sex!

329 Give yourself a hand

That's right, masturbate. Regularly. It's fun, it's free, and it'll improve your peak-ability when you're together. How? Well, you know what they say: Practice makes perfect. If you don't know how to play your own pipe organ, how do you expect *him* to figure it out? Plus, frequent Os improve below-the-belt vascularity, a measure of how quickly blood can flood the area. Translation: Keep it flowing, and it'll be a cinch to get glowing.

> **SURPRISING SEX FACT!**
>
> For men, an orgasm lasts up to 8 seconds. But for women, it can last up to 20 seconds (read it and weep, guys)!

330 Take matters into your own hands *during* lovemaking

If you took that last tip to heart and learned the best way to wet your own whistle, what's to stop you from putting those skills to good use *while* you have intercourse? There are plenty of positions that leave room for you to reach for gold while he's going at it, particularly spooning or sex from behind. Or ask him to do the honors and we'll bet he'll happily comply.

331 Build a bridge

Find it difficult to have an orgasm during intercourse? Try the "bridge" technique, in which you start with what you know works and then wean yourself from it. For example, if oral sex is your surefire ticket into orbit, have him do that until you reach the point of knowing you're going to climax within seconds. Then switch to intercourse. If all goes well, nearly anything he does at this point should light your fire. Next time, try switching to intercourse a bit sooner. Over weeks or months, your body will be able to expand its orgasmic repertoire so you can cross the finish line any way you darn please.

332 Put your foot down

Warning: If your legs are angled up during the act, you may be sabotaging your own sexual satisfaction, since this position prevents your clitoris from receiving adequate stimulation. Instead, make sure your legs are flat on the bed during the missionary position or stretched down toward his legs while you're on top. This will guarantee you're getting maximum impact right where you want it.

> > Inside the male mind

"The furrow, the gasp, the exclamation, the tightening up and then complete loosening of her muscles—it's all awesome. Orgasm is about a loss of control, and to make her lose it is a great thing."

—Ben, 29

333 Hop on top

Pore through 70 years of sex studies and you'll find that in every single one, the majority of women who reliably had orgasms during intercourse were positioned on top. Some theorize it's due to the extra control women have of their movements, others speculate it's due to the angle her pubic bone rubs against his. Or, maybe you don't care what the reason is as long as you have one, huh? So hop on!

> **SURPRISING SEX FACT!**
>
> According to a REDBOOK poll, 50 percent of women masturbate a few times a month, with 16 percent confessing they do so a few times a week and a hot-blooded 6 percent almost daily. However, a surprising 28 percent of women say they never masturbate, saying they prefer to get their jollies with their man.

334 And when you're on top, try this

Rather than merely moving your hips forward and back on one plane, imagine you're drawing an oval, with a downstroke at one end of the oval and an upstroke at the other. By taking your bump-and-grind from two dimensions to 3-D, you'll hit a lot more hot spots on you *and* him. And it looks really sensual, too.

> **SURPRISING SEX FACT!**
>
> On average, women take 27 minutes to reach their peak.

335 Add some tension

Gird your loins, girls! To bring on a Big O pronto, tense the muscles in your thighs and/or buttocks. This will bring more blood to the area, and with blood comes oxygen, and with oxygen comes breathtaking orgasms.

336 Take time-outs

If you're having intercourse and one of you is lagging behind the other on the arousal meter, take a break and switch to another activity (like oral sex or manual stimulation) that'll allow the latecomer (so to speak!) to catch up. Then, onward and upward!

337 Try the V trick

Place two fingers in the shape of a V around your privates and keep them in place during intercourse. He'll barely notice, and you'll benefit from the extra friction. You can also press down and pull up on the area, which will expose your sweet spot (your clitoris) to plenty of lusty thrusting. Enjoy!

> ## >> Inside the male mind
>
> *"I think about funerals—the casket being lowered into the ground. It's morbid, but anything that stops me from coming before my wife does is a good thing!"*
>
> *—Jay, 40*

> > Inside the male mind

"Every once in a while I have these tremendous orgasms that feel like an explosion. I call them 'screaming orgasms.'"

—Brad, 27

338 Visualize your way to an orgasm

Sure, it sounds weird, but don't knock it until you've tried it! Close your eyes and imagine that all the energy in your body is focused in two places: One, a spot slightly below your navel, is called the inner chi by devotees of Eastern erotic arts because of its proximity to the genitals. The second, the base of your spine, is considered the site of sexual energy by practitioners of Kundalini yoga. By imagining that you're holding energy in these two places, you're using the power of your mind to increase blood flow and body temperature down below—both cornerstones for a mind-boggling climax.

339 Create a "circle of fire"

If you found the visualization technique above revved your engines, wait'll you try this one. Visualize your breath as fire, then create a "circle of fire" by moving that blaze of energy through your whole body: Draw a deep, slow breath in through your nose and mouth, then push that fire breath down and feel it licking the base of your spine before you mentally release it through your genitals. This technique will really stoke your coals and convince you of the powers of positive thinking.

340 Use these four words in bed

Of course, no number of positions or techniques will catapult couples to cloud nine unless they communicate. Not a big talker in bed? These four words should get you by just fine: *faster, slower, harder,* and *softer*. Just murmur or whisper these directions and don't worry, he'll be happy to make the adjustment, especially if you follow up with an exclamation that indicates he's right on target, such as "Mmmm" or "Yes! Yes! Yes!" Or let your hands point him in the direction: Just place them on his hips or butt to control the motion so it's just how you like it.

SURPRISING SEX FACT!

According to a REDBOOK survey, 24 percent of couples have never orgasmed simultaneously with their partner, while 56 percent say they've managed to do so some of the time, and 20 percent claim it happens almost always.

>> Inside the male mind

"The Taoists say men actually die a little death when ejaculating, and I've certainly felt as if I've lost some life force. Is it like dying? No. Flying? No. More like swimming in golden-white liquid light."

—Mike, 45

341 Do *you* need to slow down? Try this

If you're one of those lucky gals who reaches orgasm too quickly for your tastes, you can put on the brakes by relaxing your body. Easier said than done? Look at your hands. Consciously try to loosen them from gripping-the-bed-sheets fists into a more tranquil pose. If your hands are relaxed, the rest of your body will follow.

342 For simultaneous Os, try the 1-to-10 game

Reaching your oh-my-God moments at the very same time is the holy grail of sex . . . and yet, all too often, couples miss the boat due to a simple misunderstanding: He interprets a certain movement or sigh as a sign you're seconds away from a tsunami, while, in fact, it means you're just warming up (women can misinterpret men's signals, too). This exercise, however, will banish all doubt. During lovemaking one night, use numbers to express how turned on both of you are, with 1 being "not at all" and 10 being "Yes, *very*." Observe which physical and verbal cues correspond with which numbers so that in the future, you'll both know exactly how close the other is—and can pace yourselves to reach the Big 10 together.

Girl talk tip-off

"Keeping my body relaxed doesn't do much for me, but if I flex my thighs while in the missionary position, I can feel an orgasm coming on pretty fast. And the tenser my body gets, the more wound up he gets, too."

—Julie, 30

343 Why stop after just one? How to shoot for multiples

We gals might not reach our peaks as quickly or as easily as men do, but there *is* one area where we have a major advantage. While men have a refractory period where they have to wait a while before having a second climax, many women can have multiple orgasms—and, as if that weren't enough good news, they can assume various forms. "Sequential multiples" are orgasms that occur two to ten minutes apart; "serial multiples" are orgasms separated by mere seconds or minutes. The trick to achieving either is simple: Keep going! Even if your first orgasm left you feeling super-sensitive, push past that. Since you're already in a heightened state of arousal (and with women, that's nine-tenths of the battle), orgasm #2 may arrive before you know it.

344 Try for a trigasm

If you thought the orgasms you were having felt good, try tripling the intensity by having him stimulate not just one, not two, but three of your hot spots at once. To do this, he stimulates your clitoris with his tongue, touches your G-spot with his finger, and strokes your anal area with another. Sure, it may take a little coordination on his part, but the results will be oh-oh-overwhelming.

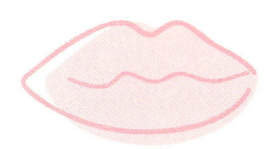

Girl talk tip-off

"Sometimes my husband and I keep our underwear on for a long time during foreplay, and I get so into it that I feel like I'm going to peak. I used to fight it so I could orgasm during sex. Now I go with it. Why stop an orgasm? My husband's so excited when I come, he never wants me to wait for him!"

—Kelly, 26

345 Repeat after us: No faking it!

We've all been there: He's trying hard, and you're trying not to yawn. True, it's tempting to put on a show and pretend you've reached your peak so you can go to sleep. But that's a bad, bad, *bad* idea, since it will seriously derail your orgasm odds in the future. Think about it: By moaning and thrashing around, you're telling him that whatever he's doing works, which would lead any logical man to try those techniques the next time, too. So, for his own sake and yours, be honest. If you think a different approach will work, tell him. If you think it's a lost cause,

SURPRISING SEX FACT!

58 percent of women have faked an orgasm at some point. And (surprise!) 28 percent of men have also, according to a REDBOOK poll.

> ### Moves men love
>
> *"When I'm on top, Kelly puts her hands firmly on my butt, letting me know how fast or slow she wants me to move. When she's ready, she pulls me deeply inside her. And her hands massage, caress, and even occasionally slap me. Talk about knowing you're in good hands!"*
>
> —Joe, 32

tell him. What are you afraid of? Unless he's got issues, he won't crumple up on the bed and cry. And if you top off your comment with "but I'd still find it a turn-on to see/hear/feel *you* come," then honestly, who'd complain?

346 Remember, an orgasm is an orgasm, no matter how it happens

Sure, reaching orgasm during intercourse is nice. But if you more easily get off during oral sex, manual stimulation, a vibrator, or some other means, please don't fall into the trap of thinking you got the consolation prize while those orgasm-during-intercourse gals hit the jackpot. Truth is, most women *don't* climax purely through hip-to-hip contact. That's just a fact, and getting bummed about it is like beating yourself up for not being able to throw a 100-mph fast ball or lift heavy furniture. So, no matter how you're having them, quit looking this gift horse in the mouth and be happy. After all, you've just had an orgasm. Enjoy it!

347 If you're about to blow, let him know

There are many reasons for this. One, so he can tell he's on track and should continue doing what he's doing. Two, so he doesn't try *changing* his technique right when you're almost there (talk about frustrating). Three, there are no sweeter words to a man's ears than these three: "I'm almost there!"

SURPRISING SEX FACT!

When REDBOOK asked women what's the maximum number of orgasms they've had during sex, 22 percent said one, 33 percent two, 27 percent three or four, and a lucky 18 percent said five or more!

CHAPTER 19

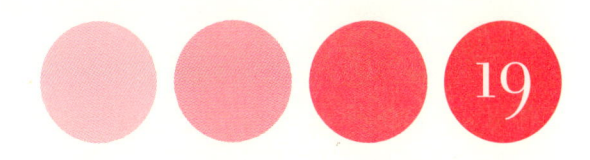

23 *very* sexy surprises

Congratulations—if you've gotten this far into this book, you're probably having some darn good sex. But over time, even the lustiest couples can start to get a little, well, comfortable . . . and that's the perfect time to shake things up with one of these shockers below. Don't worry, these bedroom bombshells don't require a ton of prep work or pushing past your kink comfort zone; sometimes just the smallest tweaks to your usual routine can amp up the electricity. So the next time you find your love life feels a little been there/done that, throw him one of these curve balls to keep him on his toes.

348   Switch the order of your usual sex steps

You know how hitting "shuffle" makes an old CD sound fresh? Same is true with sex. If you typically segue from manual stimulation to oral to intercourse, mix it up: This alone will give the sensations a whole new spin.

349   Turn on the lights

If you usually do it in the dark, shed some light on your lovemaking for an eye-opening experience (literally). Feeling bashful? Start with dim lighting or candlelight. This will reveal enough details to make you think, *Damn, look at us go!* but not so many that you start worrying, *Whoa, does he realize I haven't shaved my legs since Labor Day?*

350   Rough him up a little

Show him you're not all *that* sweet by challenging him to a wrestling match (clothing optional). Or, while having sex, lightly bite his neck or grab his butt, hard, while he's thrusting. It won't take much to make him think, *Hel-lo, who's this?*

351   Rent something racy

Tonight, DVD stands for Daring Vixen Device: Let him believe you've picked up a standard blockbuster. Pop it in, then express shock and indignation as the stars of *Night Shift Nurses* or *Horny Happy Hour* start shagging nonstop. "That's not what I ordered!" you say indignantly. "But, since we paid for it . . ."

352 Set your own personal sex record

One time, two times, three times—and again. See just how many times you can do it in one day. Discover hidden wells of endurance, creativity, and orgasmability you never knew you had—and swap high fives afterward.

353 Throw in a few road signs

Take an eyeliner pencil and write "Kiss me" or "Caress me" on your stomach, breast or other body part, adding arrows to tell him where to go (and what to do) next. Not only will he be sweetly surprised when you disrobe, but you'll get exactly what you want, where you want it!

354 Savor a novel sensation

Rather than dwelling on how fantastic sex feels or looks, tune into how it tastes. Kiss and lick your way from head to toe and take note of the different flavors. Is his neck salty? Is his inner elbow slightly sweet? Or buy a few kinds of flavored body lotion (try the Motion Lotion Sampler Pack, goodvibes.com), rub them on different parts of your body, and play Guess That Flavor: Is it banana? Wild cherry? Triggering your taste buds will turn sex into even more of a multisensory experience.

> **SURPRISING SEX FACT!**
>
> According to a REDBOOK poll, 74 percent of couples occasionally turn the light on when having sex; 9 percent say they're *usually* on!

One woman's sex secret—revealed

"It doesn't matter how tired I am; if my husband pops in porn, I'll wake up and watch. It's the fastest and easiest way to jump-start my libido."

—Fran, 40

355 Pounce in the middle of the night

No doubt about it, sex at 3 a.m. feels different. Impulsive. Furtive. Dreamlike. And *definitely* surprising, at least as far as he's concerned!

356 Stick to the shallow end

Instead of diving right in, throw him for a loop next time by starting with short, shallow thrusts before you let him go deep. This will hit the most sensitive spots on you (the opening of the vagina) and him (the head of the penis) and drive you both crrr-azy.

SURPRISING SEX FACT!

33 percent of couples have called in "sick" to work so they could spend the day in bed together, according to a REDBOOK survey.

357 Play hooky together

Calling in sick to work when you're anything but will give you a big bad adrenaline rush, and having the house to yourselves for out-in-the-open action will make you feel like nooky-crazed newlyweds. No one at your office need be the wiser.

358 Turn up the temperature . . .

Make love in the sun's warm rays by a window where the light streams in. Or get physical on a rug in front of a roaring fire. Or, if it's summertime, just turn off your air conditioner. As your body becomes flushed, your nerves become more sensitive to touch. And, of course, the only thing more stunning than bare skin is bare skin bathed in a gleaming sheen of sweat—all of which will add a whole new kind of heat to your close encounter.

Girl talk tip-off

"When it's dark, my husband and I are operating purely by touch, and that can limit how well you read each other's sexual signals. When the lights are on, I can tell when he likes a certain way I've touched him, and I can make a mental note to do it again."

—Jane, 37

359 . . . Or turn it down

Come one cold winter night, turn down the thermostat in your bedroom (it's good for the environment, after all), snuggle under the covers, and create some of your own heat. The refreshing contrast between the cool air and your warm bodies will give you goose bumps . . . in a good way.

360 Challenge him to the world's quickest quickie

Ready, set, go!

361 Stay joined at the hip when he least expects it

This move is bound to impress and make you feel powerful. Whether you're on top, on the bottom, or somewhere in between, seamlessly switch sex positions without interrupting the action by wrapping your legs around his waist, throwing your arms around his shoulders, and rolling over in unison.

One woman's sex secret—revealed

"Porn and taping ourselves doing it all add to the adrenaline of sex and create a very open dialogue of intimacy and trust. I could not talk about these things with someone I didn't deeply trust."

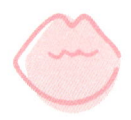

—Carey, 30

Girl talk tip-off

"The other night my husband and I moved so we could make love right under the ceiling fan. The air on our exposed bodies felt so amazing. Next time we're going to try turning it on high."

—Jennifer, 31

362 During intercourse, switch to oral sex

Then switch back. Alternating sensations will make each one even more exhilarating.

363 Make love to the camera

Sure, digital camcorders are great for filming Junior's first birthday. But admit it, they're also great for recording you and your guy in some *very* compromising positions. For the sexiest results, heed these tips from porn producer Candida Royalle: Nix harsh overhead lights and turn on lamps, which cast much more flattering light. And since handheld shots will look shaky, set the camera on a table or nightstand close enough so that your body fills the frame (because what's the fun if you can't see what's going on?). And no matter how much you enjoy the missionary position, keep in mind it doesn't offer much eye candy. Woman on top, sex from behind, or spooning will all provide a much better view for you to both enjoy later.

364   Keep your hands on the move

During sex, instead of parking your hands on his shoulders or the small of his back, vow to keep your fingertips roaming. The extrasensory input will supersize your pleasure—and his.

365   Try the Spiral of Nines

For a dizzying new spin on the old in-and-out, try this ancient erotic technique. Have him start with nine quick, shallow thrusts, then do one slow, deep thrust, followed by eight shallow ones, two deep ones, and so on until he reaches nine deep thrusts. Then reverse until you're caterwauling like crazed opera singers. What makes this move so exhilarating is its yin-yang balance of variety and predictability: You experience a range of sensations, but it builds in a rhythm you can anticipate and look forward to. Yes, it takes discipline. But consider it the black belt of sex: If you pull it off, you're a master!

366   Fan the flames of your desire

You might not have seen the movie *Body Heat*, but as the name implies, it's a scorcher. Go Hollywood at home with a cue from this '80s film noir by getting busy in front of a fan. Think thin, rippling sheets, billowing

> **SURPRISING SEX FACT!**
>
> According to a REDBOOK survey, 62 percent of couples claim they've had sex at their in-laws' house. Guess it's a thrill trying to be sneaky so mom and dad don't hear!

One woman's sex secret—revealed

"Sometimes when I see the sweat running down my husband's chest and onto my body, I think, Wow, look at us go!"

—Tanya, 30

hair, your hot, sweaty bodies awash in cool blasts of air . . . we get breathless just thinking about it.

367 Do it on deadline

Set an egg timer next to the bed. Tell him he gets to pleasure you for 10 minutes. When the buzzer goes off, you return the favor. Racing against time will get your heart racing, giving you added sexual momentum.

368 Get it on in front of a mirror

Those playboys from the '70s had mirrors over their waterbeds for a reason: Watching yourself make love is unbelievably arousing. No need to install a ceiling mirror; try simply propping one up at the foot of the bed. Then try these positions: him seated facing the mirror, with you sitting on his lap facing forward as well, gives you both an eyeful of the action below; doggy style, using the mirror to hold each other's gaze and up the intimacy. Even a small hand mirror can lend a fresh perspective to your usual activities. Use one during oral sex, for instance, and the view from down under will astonish and amaze.

369 Share a steamy bedtime story

Even if you've rented plenty of porn and flipped through a slew of racy magazines together, here's one form of sexual entertainment you probably *haven't* tried yet: erotic audiobooks. Search for and download titillating tracks at audible.com; if kids may be listening in, get a headphone splitter so you can both plug in in private. Rarely are your ears the focus of so much sexual input—and, unlike more visual forms of stimulation, audio leaves plenty to the imagination. Let the sounds carry you into another world.

370 Check into a motel

Just think: Tons of fun, none of the cleanup. Yes, a change of scenery could do you well, indeed.

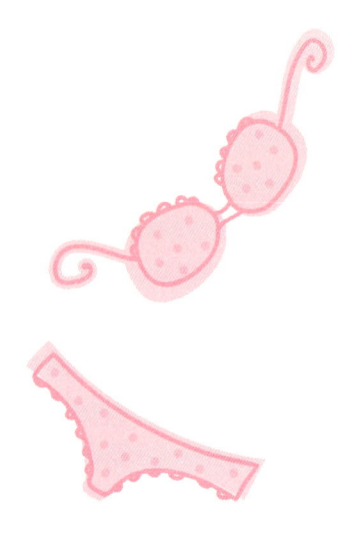

CHAPTER 20

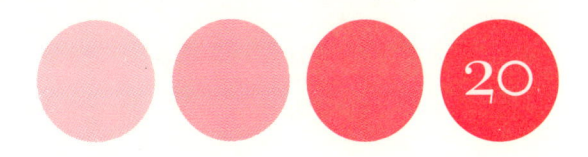

Sex toys: What's the buzz?

Way back in the 1880s, some lucky maiden somewhere volunteered to roadtest an odd-looking device that would revolutionize sex as we know it: the very first vibrator. Within seconds of placing it on her genitals, boom, she was in orbit—and boy, have we come a long way since then. Today, there is an infinite array of sex toys available. Some look like bunnies, or come with a remote; one even plugs into your iPod (no joke). But which one is right for you? And what if your sweetie freaks when he sees it? Whether you've yet to give in to the buzz and buy one or have worn out a whole manufacturing line's worth and are looking for the next great gadget, consider this chapter your guide to exploring everything today's technology has to offer.

Curious about sex toys, but have questions or concerns? Then read on . . .

371 Don't worry, vibrators *won't* dull your nerves

Many women worry that a vibrator's strong stimulatory powers will desensitize their nerve endings, making them less responsive over time. But nerves just don't work like that. True, continuous stimulation may numb an area somewhat (which is why you should move your vibrator around on your genitals—you can't expect it to do *all* the work!). But no matter how much of a pounding they get, nerves bounce back within minutes as good as new. So don't worry, you can have as many toygasms as you darn well please without paying some Karmic price down the road.

372 Not sure what vibrator to get?

Which vibrator you should get depends on your needs. To find the right one, consider the following:

- **Do you want a sex toy for clitoral or vaginal stimulation, or both?**
  Smaller ones are usually just for the clitoris.
- **Do you want one that's plug-in or battery-operated?**
  Plug-ins are more of a pain, but they're also powerful and won't run out of juice at an inopportune moment.
- **What kind of vibes do you like—strong or faint? Fast or slow?**
  If you're not sure, get one with various settings. When in doubt, swallow your pride and ask the sales staff for

suggestions. These days, there are plenty of female-friendly establishments that can perkily discuss the pros and cons of various models. Or go online to goodvibes.com or babeland.com.

> ## SURPRISING SEX FACT!
>
> A study from the Berman Center in Chicago found that 55 percent of women in relationships use vibrators; only 34 percent of single women do the same.

373 Convinced he won't go for it? Broach the topic this way

Guys dig gadgets—no shocker there—so he'll probably be thrilled to bring one to bed. Still, he may wonder, *Does this mean my own skills aren't up to snuff?* To dispel his fears, steer clear of any comments that suggest you're fixing a problem, like, "I'm not having an orgasm with you, so I guess it's time to get us one of those sex toys and see if *that'll* do the job." Instead, present it as the icing on the cake of your love life by saying, "I'm thinking maybe it would be fun to experiment. How about we try a sex toy?" If he balks, remind him that sex toys are usually used on the clitoris

---

Girl talk tip-off

"Toys deliver incredible sensations. Why not use the latest technology to make sex more stimulating?"

—Judy, 30

versus inserted vaginally, so there'll be plenty of room for him. To further keep him from feeling sidelined, consider handing the controls over to him with a coy, "Why don't you try it on me?" This will reinforce the idea that *he's* making you come, and that the toy is merely an accessory. Trust us, once he sees it in action, he'll come around and start enjoying his newfound freedom. After all, making a woman come takes effort—and you've just lightened his workload.

374 There is no such thing as "vibrator addiction"

Sure, sex toys feel good, but that doesn't mean women are at risk of becoming so dependent that they spend their days holed up in their apartment, alone, until friends stage an intervention. The grain of truth in this myth is that women *can* get so accustomed to the ease and speed of having an orgasm this way that they start itching to reach for it *every* time they have sex. If this happens to you, all you need to do is ask yourself: What's your rush? Reaching Kingdom Come through intercourse, oral or manual stimulation may take a little longer, but unless the kids are on their way home or *American Idol* starts in five minutes, there's no reason you can't take your time and appreciate getting off the old-fashioned way.

> **SURPRISING SEX FACT!**
>
> The vibrator was initially used by doctors in the late 19th century to cure women of hysteria. All we can say is, thank god we don't have to book a doctor's appointment to get off anymore!

Curious which toys you'll enjoy? Consider these popular options...

375   The Hitachi Magic Wand

The first thing you'll think when you see it is *Holy cow, it's huge!* Don't worry, this foot-long, plug-in contraption isn't meant for insertion (although you can purchase attachments that are). Just place the tip on your privates and you'll see why in this case, bigger is better: This sucker packs some powerful vibes (if it's *too* much, wrap it in bed sheets). It's not exactly sexy-looking, but that can be a plus; anyone who spots it will assume it's your typical back massager. If only they knew.

376   The Rabbit

Yup, it's got cute little eyes, ears, and a nose that, um, wiggles in a way your nether regions will enjoy. Plus it's designed to hit your clitoris *and* your vagina at the same time for twice the kicks.

377   The Pocket Rocket

True to its name, this lipstick-size vibrator can be easily stashed in your purse or luggage for on-the-go fun.

378   The Butterfly

This toy is one you wear rather than wield, leaving your hands (and his) free to wander and cause trouble elsewhere. How's that for easy?

379 Remote-Control Butterfly

You wear it, he mans the controls and drives you crazy turning it on and off at whim. Some models are even so quiet you can wear them out on the town, if you dare.

380 Vibrating Cock Ring

Worn around the base of his penis, this device can turn intercourse into an orgasmfest, since every thrust will feel extra tingly. (Bonus: He gets to enjoy the buzz, too.)

381 The OhMiBod

We highly doubt Apple ever factored *this* into a five-year business plan, but nonetheless, this vibrator plugs into your iPod and—get this—pulses to the beat of whatever song you're listening to. Rock on!

CHAPTER 21

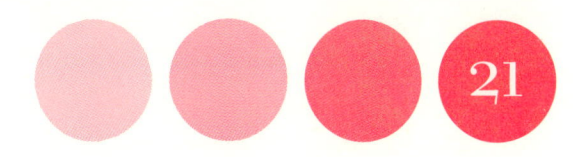

You wanna have sex *where*?!

You've heard stories of people who've done it. Maybe you've even thought about trying it yourself. Still, you've got questions: Is it safe? Is it fun? Is it legal? Whether the "it" you're referring to is sex on an airplane, beach, the boss's desk, a moving car, or some other exciting yet questionable locale, we understand why you're curious: Because the view of your bedroom ceiling can get old after a while. Because trying out places where you could get caught is exciting. Because new venues offer new challenges (ever try it in a hammock?), new sensations (mmmm, Jacuzzi jets), and new experiences you can nudge each other and giggle about. So, wherever the mood strikes, we've got the info you need to pull it off with panache—and without mosquito bites, sand in crevices, security cameras, or other unwelcome distractions.

To have sex on a beach . . .

382 Slather on sunscreen

Sure, beaches seem like idyllic spots for some lovin', but beware: The sun's rays will fry pasty white nether flesh in no time. So stay in the shade under your umbrella or make sure you've swathed all the necessary body parts in SPF 2000.

383 Drink up

The longer you work up a sweat, the bigger the risk of dehydration or sunstroke, so make sure to have plenty of fluids handy (and piña coladas don't count, since alcohol is a diuretic that will only speed the dehydration process).

384 Keep sand out of crevices

Getting grains of sand in your nether nooks and crannies can be a huge buzzkill, so lay down a beach towel before your romp or set up camp near the surf, where the sand is wet and compact and less likely to fly right where you don't want it.

SURPRISING SEX FACT!

Other than the bed, where are couples most likely to get it on? According to a REDBOOK survey, 44 percent said in their living room, 28 percent in the shower, 25 percent on the floor, and 3 percent on the kitchen table.

On a plane...

385 Use discretion

This sexual exploit's considered so impressive they've got a whole club named after it, but does becoming a Mile-High Member put you at risk for arrest? Well, think about it this way: Most airlines would probably prefer to avoid the embarrassing publicity that could come with dragging you off their plane in handcuffs. All in all, flight attendants use their discretion with onboard hookups, usually asking passengers to discontinue behaviors that might make others uncomfortable. So if you're going to risk it, do it in the lavatory instead of in your seat, be quiet, be quick, and most people will look the other way.

386 Time it right

The last thing you want is a long line of passengers who need to pee giving you dirty looks. So plan your tryst when bathroom traffic is low; red-eye flights are ideal. It's best if one of you enters the bathroom a couple minutes before the other, and stagger your return to your seats as well.

387 Try these positions

It's no shock that teeny-tiny airplane bathrooms aren't optimal for lovemaking—they hardly accommodate *one* body, let alone two. For maximum maneuverability, stand with one leg on the toilet with your man embracing you from behind. Rumor has it that the low atmospheric pressure can increase the intensity of an orgasm, so stay tuned for quite a finale!

In a Jacuzzi . . .

388   Keep hygiene in mind

Sure, shagging in a hot tub is so '70s sexy. But be warned, strange things *can* grow in the warm bubbly water. Public hot tubs, if not well maintained, can harbor bacteria that can lead to *pseudomonas folliculitis*, a skin infection that causes an itchy rash that must be treated with antibiotics. So, swim—and *ahem*—at your own risk, or stick to privately owned tubs.

389   Birth control may also be compromised

Don't rely on condoms, spermicides, diaphragms, or contraceptive sponges for birth control, caution experts, as their effectiveness in hot tubs is unstudied. Plus, condoms can deteriorate in hot water and be notoriously hard to put (and keep) on. So if pregnancy isn't on your agenda, use other forms of birth control, like the Pill.

390   Choose the right lube

Hot water can make lubricants—natural and otherwise—dissolve more quickly, causing extra friction and tender, raw skin. To avoid the ouch factor, get a silicone-based lube, which is water-resistant and will keep the good times rolling.

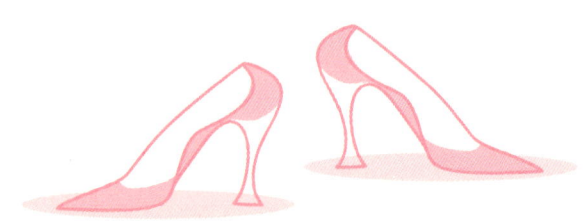

391 Ride them jets

Place your privates in line with those warm pulses of water and watch out—many women find the sensation very stimulating, and the perfect way to warm up for the main event. The easiest position for intercourse is if he sits and you straddle his lap—that way, you can both keep your heads well above water.

In the shower . . .

392 Two words: rubber mat

Without it, chances are high that you'll slip, grab your shower curtain and tear it off its hanger, conk your head on a tiled wall, or worse. Don't risk it. It's a small investment with big benefits (read: traction).

393 Kill the harsh lights

Sure, those 100-watt bulbs are fantastic for applying eyeliner or ferreting out blackheads. But right now, that level of detail could be a mood killer. Use candles instead.

394 Clean him up before you get dirty

To let him know this won't be your typical wash-'n'-go, stand behind him, soap yourself up, then wrap your arms around his chest and press your breasts against his back. Wrap one soapy leg around his and swivel your body up and down to *really* create some suds. Carefully switch legs and repeat. Next, turn him around and treat him to the same soapy swivel front to front. We think he'll take the hint!

395 Don't use soap as a stand-in for lube

If you find yourself in need of extra lubrication for manual stimulation or for intercourse, *don't* reach for the soap or the shampoo. Prolonged use of these substances on delicate areas (and your genitals definitely qualify) will cause the skin there to dry and crack like the Sahara. So stick to lubes that are meant for this purpose, like Astroglide, K-Y Jelly or, better yet, silicone, which is water-resistant.

396 Try these positions

For maximum stability that will keep the spray out of your face, have him stand behind you and take you from behind as you lean forward to prop yourself against the shower wall. If you're in a tub, you can also raise one leg and prop one foot on the lip for easier access. Or face each other and hook one leg around his waist, resting your hand flat on the shower wall behind you to steady yourself.

> **SURPRISING SEX FACT!**
>
> According to a REDBOOK survey, 67 percent of you have had sex in a car. But we don't care how good a driver you are, accidents happen—especially when you're joined at the hip and hurtling forward at 65 miles per hour. So don't do it while driving.

In the great outdoors...

397 Don't let the bugs bite

Birds twittering, sunlight streaming through dappled foliage . . . no doubt, going wild in a forest or field sounds idyllic. But Mother Nature does have its downsides. For one: mosquitoes. To avoid getting big itchy welts in all the wrong places, don't wear perfumes or scented lotions, which attract insects in swarms. Bring a blanket to avoid ground-dwelling creepy crawlies and a waterproof jacket or sleeping bag to keep morning dew or recent rainfall from turning your romp into a mud-wrestling match.

398 Maintain some privacy

In case nosy hikers stumble across your tryst saying, "Hel-*lo*, what have we here?" dress for easy access with clothes that can stay on for the whole ride, like a skirt or sundress sans underwear and a front-hook bra. The best position to avoid detection is lying sideways facing each other, with a blanket over you. That way, in case anyone is peeping through their binocs from afar, it'll look like you're merely snuggling (as if).

In the car...

399 Park it—in these positions

You've pulled into Lookout Point and are ready to pounce like hormonal teenagers. But first, get your butt out of the driver's seat in case your impassioned flailing results in a jarring elbow-on-horn honk. Instead, straddle him in the passenger seat or move to the back for some missionary action (probably most easily accomplished with your legs up rather than lying flat; he can also kneel on the floor).

400   Do it *on* the car instead of in it

It's every guy's dream to christen the hood of his car, so why not humor him? The next time you're headed somewhere you're in no rush to get to, entice him into a detour with, "Why don't we just go for a ride right here?" Then sit your tush on the hood and wrap your legs around his waist, or stand facing the windshield and lean waaay over as he takes you from behind. Even in the privacy of your garage, it's hot, and he'll be in heaven.

401   Added bonus: Get frisky while you're washing it

"Accidentally" spray yourself—and him—while wearing a white T-shirt and congratulations, you've just staged your own wet-T-shirt contest! And let's face it: No matter how sophisticated your guy is, there's something about his girl in a clingy, see-through tee that will get his attention like never before. You'll be his spring break come to life!

On a waterbed . . .

402   Remember, water is . . . watery

Sure, bumping and grinding on a surface that undulates along with you may seem groovy in theory, but the lack of firm footing can present challenges. Probably the least waterbed-friendly position is sex from behind, since having all your weight on six points (four knees and two hands) can put a lot of pressure on the mattress and make for a wobbly ride. You're better off in positions that distribute weight evenly, like missionary or side by side.

403   Get a grip

Since a waterbed gives when you push, thrusting may lack its usual oomph. If you find the surface a little *too* yielding, though, all is not lost. Waterbed *frames* are usually constructed out of wood or metal, so inch over to the edge and wedge your toes along the lip or grab it with your hands to go at it with more gusto.

In a hammock...

404   Get yourself a quality model

Brazilians have been sleeping and procreating in them for centuries, so obviously it *is* possible . . . only how? First, go for a cotton style if you can; ones made of rope or nylon will be mighty uncomfortable. Also make sure it's well anchored and knotted to the wall or tree, since the only thing more painful than falling out of a hammock is doing so with someone on top of you.

405   Rock this way

Feel trapped like two flies in a web? Angle your bodies more diagonally, with your head and feet toward the sides. This will cause the hammock to flatten out a bit and give you a little more wiggle room. But still, it won't be much, which means your best bets position-wise are spooning or woman on top. Or, even better, kick him out so he can stand or kneel next to you and use that natural rocking motion to his advantage.

At the office . . .

406 Wait until late-night hours

After all, it's far safer to risk getting caught by Mr. Janitor than the Boss Man. And besides, if you're working into the wee hours, you almost deserve to misbehave a little, don'tcha think?

407 Check for security cameras

Beware, many offices have 24-hour surveillance—especially in storage rooms where theft might be a problem (and sex seems all too tempting). So, scan before you strip.

408 Use desks to your advantage

Whether you have your eye on the head honcho's mahogany monolith or your more modest workstation, all desks are waist height—perfect for quick hip-to-hip contact with you seated on the edge and him standing in front of you. Or, if risk of a walk-in is high, consider scooting under the desk and going down on him while he's seated. You'll feel like a bombshell secretary from a '40s detective film, and any coworker passing by will think, "My, Kirk really enjoys poring over those spreadsheets, doesn't he?"

CHAPTER 22

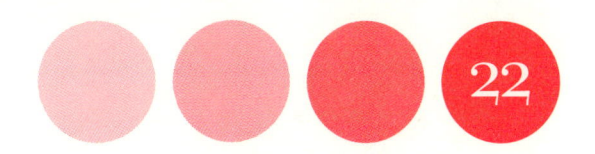

The shy girl's guide to speaking up in bed

For the most part, it's all but impossible to shut us gals up. We gab for hours with our girlfriends, explain in painstaking detail how we want our couch reupholstered, and are masters at coaxing men out of their shells. But once the lights dim and the clothes come off, something weird happens: We become tongue-tied. Deep down, we know most men love hearing some blush-worthy verbal feedback. But how do you get started if it doesn't come naturally, and what the heck should you say? Allow us to help you loosen those vocal chords and add some fine audio effects to your lovemaking. Being verbal is the best way there is to get your guy in tune with your needs, explore his own, and build a whole new level of romantic rapport.

409   Start simple

First off, keep in mind that you don't need to swear like a sailor to get your point across. In bed, just about anything you say will carry an erotic charge, so if you're on the bashful side, try these easy openers: If he's doing something you like, try saying/whispering/purring, "That feels good" or "Yes, there." Once you're comfortable with those, work up to "Mmm, it feels so good when you _____" [fill in the blank]. Sounds tame, but if you're the silent type, just a few words can pack quite a punch. Plus there's an added benefit: These appreciative remarks also clue him in to which moves he's doing work for you, thus guaranteeing plenty of repeat performances.

410   Plagiarize from professionals

Want to whisper something saucy but are drawing a blank on what to say? That, dear readers, is where porn magazines or erotica (such as Susie Bright's *The Best American Erotica* anthologies) can help. Every page is flush with material; feel free to borrow a few bon mots and try them out for size in bed. Or read a whole chapter together in bed one night (out loud, of course). Don't be surprised if your randy reading inspires you to act out what you're hearing.

411   Use words *you* find a turn-on

No doubt you're aware that there are countless colorful ways to describe his anatomy, and yours, and the various ways you can fit them together. So you should never feel cornered into saying something crass if that's not your style; just pick from the many less-offensive alternatives that you *do* find arousing. For example, maybe you prefer "breast" over "boob," or "go down on me" over more graphic options. Don't worry, he won't be picky, and will get a rise out of anything you say.

412 Rehearse your lines a little

Once you've found a few titillating turns of phrase you'd like to say to your guy, that doesn't mean you'll automatically be able to trot them out in bed. Stage fright can still take hold, so it's best if you practice saying them when you're alone (very alone, we might add). Trust us, saying, "Put your hands on my [bleep]" the twentieth time won't make you wince like it might have at first. Or try talking dirty the next time you're masturbating, so you start to subconsciously link sexual arousal with your sultry sound effects.

413 Describe what you're doing—or going to do

If you're ever at a loss for what to say, this fallback will always fill the silence: Like a sportscaster, keep a running commentary on the action ("Now I'm stroking your chest, now I'm kissing your stomach, now . . . "). Or explain what's ahead ("Next, I'm going to lick your . . . "). Bonus: You'll build a sexy sense of anticipation for what's to come.

> ### Moves men love
>
> "Occasionally she'll page me and send the message 'I want to [bleep] tonight.' I love getting playful, devilish little notes like this. It lets me know that she's going to be ready and raring to go when I get home."
>
> —Paul, 27

414 Make it a two-way conversation by asking questions

Think your guy would like to join in with a few not-so-sweet nothings but doesn't know how? Make it easy for him by asking him questions. Ask, "Does that feel good?" (even the shyest guys should be able to respond with "God, yes!"), and once he's comfortable answering yes/no questions, try a more open-ended query, like "What would you like me to kiss/lick/stroke next?" or "What would you like to do to me?" All too soon, you'll have a dirty talk duet going on.

415 Invent your own sexy slang

For extra originality points, consider coining your own love lingo that encapsulates sexual techniques or positions that get your blood pumping. Here's a failproof formula: Start with "the." Add an adjective that applies to small animals, such as "frisky." Finish with the name of a wild animal, like "gazelle." Look out! You crazy kids do The Frisky Gazelle . . . and can request it at whim.

416 Remember, it's not just what you say, but how you say it

When it comes to talking dirty, delivery is everything. And your options are endless: Say it a few notes higher (or lower) than usual. Whisper it. Sigh it. Moan it. Growl it. And if you don't give a crap about the neighbors, shout it! Each will bring out a very different side of your sexual personality, from breathless baby doll to take-charge tigress. It'll also show Mr. Smarty Pants there's a lot about you he hasn't figured out yet!

417 Let loose when he least expects it

Talk dirty in bed and he's one happy man. Talk dirty *out* of bed, and he won't be able to think straight until he can drag you back there. Plant a scandalous comment in the middle of a mundane moment—i.e., "I can't wait to get in your pants once we're done loading this dishwasher"—and your naughty non sequitur will win you double bad-girl points. And since he may not be able to ravish you immediately, it'll only serve to amp up his anticipation.

418 Compliments can be dirty talk, too

Next time you're both naked, pick a part of his body that's your favorite and praise it to the skies. Start with "You've got the most beautiful shoulders/chest/butt I've ever seen," then expand by adding how it makes you feel (safe? weak-kneed? just plain turned on?). This works wonders on men because they rarely receive flattery on their appearance, so when they do, it serves double duty as dirty talk *and* an ego inflator.

Girl talk tip-off

"I reminisce about the last time my husband and I had great sex—his touch, his breath on my skin, his sweet murmurings in my ear. By focusing on my sexiest memories, I'll bring myself to a fired-up state that often leads us into bed."

—Sasha, 36

419 Try some long-distance dirty talk

Call him and say you can't wait until he gets home so you can [fill in the blank]. Rest assured, your phone foreplay will guarantee he'll hightail it back in no time.

420 Have some 1-900 fun

While he's watching TV in the living room, call him from the bedroom on your cell phone and tell him that you're touching yourself. Describe exactly what you're doing—and what you're longing for him to do to you. Then invite him to join you in the bedroom (if he isn't there already!).

421 Put it in writing

Yup, recording your racy thoughts on paper counts as dirty talk, too. So slip a note in his pocket or briefcase saying, "Right now, I'm thinking about your sexy shoulders/smile/butt and wishing you were here." Or send him a suggestive e-mail or IM message: "You, me, the bedroom, 10 p.m." Drive him wild by logging off before he can write back begging for delicious details.

> ## >> Inside the male mind
>
> *"She called me at work and told me that she couldn't stop thinking about me and that I had to come home—at once. Sensing I was in for more than my usual welcome-home kiss, I rushed to get there. The anticipation that built during my commute was agonizing and only made me that much more excited when I arrived home to find her waiting in bed."* —Michael, 30

CHAPTER 23

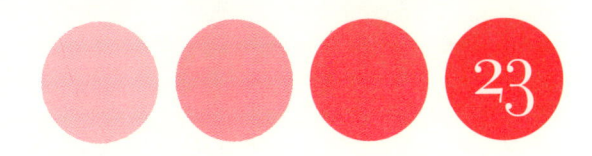

Fantasies: His, yours, and how to make them come true (if you want to)

Admit it: Buried deep within the recesses of your mind lies a collection of flickering images and steamy plot lines that turn you on. A lot. And yet, for all the enjoyment we get out of these private musings, rarely do we reveal them to others—not even to the loving, trusting, and *very* curious guy lying next to us in bed (don't worry, he's probably equally chicken).

No doubt about it, putting your secret desires out there can be scary no matter how well you know each other. But that's all the more reason to share them, since they'll reveal entirely new facets of yourselves to each other, provide fresh fodder for real-life adventures, and can help you both feel known, loved, and accepted on a new level. So, if you're *ready* to take a virtual vacation for two to the adult playground of Let's Pretend, here's your ticket. First, we'll show you how to discuss your fantasies, then we'll show you how to act them out if you're so inclined. Whatever you do, you're in for quite a trip.

How to talk about your fantasies...

> ### SURPRISING SEX FACT!
>
> According to the *Psychological Bulletin*, 82 percent of women and 84 percent of men say they have sexual fantasies during intercourse; 74 percent of women (and 100 percent of men) say they fantasize while masturbating.

422 Put him at ease

First, make it clear you won't frown, laugh, or freak out if he reveals a turn-on that's a little off the beaten path. Create a "safe zone" by saying, "I want you to know that in this bed, there is no right or wrong. No matter what you say, I won't judge you." This carte blanche will make it easier to open up.

423 Manage his expectations

Just because you're sharing your private reveries doesn't mean you'll be breaking out the necessary props any time soon, or at all. Since your guy can assume that's the direction you're going, say, "This doesn't mean I'll be up for doing it. But hearing it would be a real turn-on." Many men feel exactly the same way, and are content to talk about a racy bondage fantasy but still have sex as usual.

424 Ask him what fantasies he has about *you*

When starting out, it's best to avoid open-ended queries like "What are your fantasies?" Not only does it put him on the spot, but he might also blurt out something scary—like he has the hots

> > Inside the male mind

"I think about the scene from True Lies *when Jamie Lee Curtis dances for Arnold Schwarzenegger, Meg Ryan faking an orgasm in* When Harry Met Sally, *and Kelly McGillis and Tom Cruise in her four-poster bed with satin all over in* Top Gun."

— Doug, 37

for your best friend. (Rule of thumb: Never ask a question you're not prepared to hear the answer to.) Instead, try, "Do you ever fantasize about us? What are we doing?" This way, he can share some safer musings. (And remember, this goes both ways, so don't go blurting out how cute his boss is unless you're looking for a fight.)

425   Talk about sexy sensations

If you don't feel comfortable describing a specific scene, try talking about sexy sensations: the feel of his strong hands on your body, his warm breath on your neck, the enveloping mild breeze on your last beach vacation that made you feel relaxed and sensual. We're programmed to think fantasizing means hitting

> > Inside the male mind

"Sometimes I think about past lovers. I've even imagined one coworker naked (if only she knew)."

—Michael, 35

> > Inside the male mind

"I picture me and my wife at a swingers party, having sex while others watch, or her and another woman going down on me, or her and me servicing a woman."

—Mike, 42

"play" on some hot scene like the pizza delivery boy and the oversexed housewife. But oftentimes, it's much simpler—that doesn't mean it shouldn't get air time.

426 Give him options

If he's tongue-tied, treat him to a game of multiple choice with questions like, "What would turn you on: me dressed up as a nurse, a schoolgirl, or in head-to-toe leather?" He'll be able to reveal his preferences without implying that he's unhappy with what you've currently got going in bed.

SURPRISING SEX FACT!

18 percent of women fantasize about having sex with more than one man at a time; 33 percent of men fantasize about having sex with more than one woman at a time, according to the *Psychological Bulletin*.

> ## >> Inside the male mind
>
> *"I fantasize about my wife doing things she won't, or things I don't want to tell her I want, like anal sex or role play."*
>
> —Dave, 41

427   Lead him in with examples

Ready to hear the racier stuff in his noggin? It may feel safer for both of you to start by talking about someone *else's* steamy vision—a scene in a movie you watched, an erotic book you read, that "friend of a friend" who's dabbling in S&M. Say, "I can't stop thinking about that threesome scene in the movie *Henry & June*. I thought it was a turn-on, did you?" It's easier for a guy to say, "I like that" than confessing to his own fantasy out of thin air. From there, you can easily get more personal with questions like "So, do you ever fantasize about that?"

428   Ask him to elaborate

Once you know the gist of his fantasy, this is where the fun *really* begins: Get him to spill all the juicy details by asking questions. If, say, he fantasizes about having sex with you and another woman, ask "What does she look like?" or "I can't quite see her lips, where are they on your body?" If he's too shy to fill in the blanks, ask him if he'd like you to pitch in your two cents. (Rule of thumb on the threesome scenario: Make the woman your physical opposite. If you're small breasted give her dizzying cleavage; if you're all-American make her exotic.) Whatever scene you weave, it's bound to get you both hot and bothered.

> > Inside the male mind

"I never fantasize about being with another woman. When I'm kissing my wife on the lips, I'm fantasizing about kissing her on her lips, or somewhere else. If I'm kissing her somewhere else, I may fantasize about kissing her on the lips."

—Timothy, 45

429 Pen a tale of passion

If you're more of a writer than a talker, weaving fantasies can still be a collaborative effort. Here's how: Write down a few lines of your fantasy on a piece of paper, then pass it to your guy. He writes a few more sentences building off your scenario, then passes it back so you can write some more, and so on and so on. The plot twists in your tale speak volumes about what whets your sexual appetites. Plus, by the end (and this can take weeks or months if the hero and/or heroine of your story continue discovering new turn-ons) you've got *quite* a keepsake on your hands, huh?

430 Thank him for sharing

Whatever he says, reward his efforts with a "Thank you, I feel much closer to you." Don't feel compelled to make his fantasies come true; your goal is to share, not put on a one-act play—unless you want to, of course. If so, go for it! More on that next.

How to make your fantasies come true . . .

431 Be his genie in a bottle

Tonight, grant him one sexual wish. Naturally, you reserve final veto power, but you're still giving him plenty of room to let his imagination run wild.

432 Try this card trick

To get a full gander of the possibilities you two could explore, buy a pack of three-by-five-inch cards. Each of you jot down one of your fantasies per card. Use as many cards as you like, and don't worry about whether it's politically correct, easy to act out in real life, or even if your partner will like it. Then reveal your cards to each other. As you do, divide them into three piles: fantasies you want to become real (i.e., sex on a secluded beach), fantasies you'd rather keep that way (such as

One woman's sex secret—revealed

"I was scared to suggest we share our secret sexual thoughts. I didn't have those racy scenarios of dirty doctor and innocent nurse or the lusty librarian, and it made me feel so tame. One night, though, I started dreamily saying to my husband, 'Wouldn't it be so nice if we were in a cabana on some tropical island . . .' and he picked it up with something like, 'and our skin is so warm and toasty and I kiss you under the sun.' We both added lines to the tale, creating such a sensual, sexy story that it got us both fired up."

—Christine, 34

a threesome), and fantasies that aren't up one person's alley (sure, doing it dressed up as sports team mascots might not be your thing, but remember, no judgments). Discard the third pile, but keep the rest. Then, the next time you're up for an adventure, have one partner pick from the deck of possibilities. If you choose a fantasy you want to keep that way, discuss it in detail during lovemaking. If you choose a fantasy you want to act out, do what you can to make it come true!

Does bondage get you hot? Then try these tips . . .

433 Start simple

Pinning his hands over his head, behind his back, or just ordering him to "not move an inch until I'm done with you" or "not come until I tell you to" will create sexy sensations of

> **SURPRISING SEX FACT!**
>
> According to a study by the *Psychological Bulletin*, only 32 percent of women and 26 percent of men say that their partners are aware of their sexual fantasies. Maybe it's because 24 percent of women and 31 percent of men feel guilty about having them in the first place. Open up, though, and you might find that your fears are unfounded . . . and feel accepted in a whole new way.

> ### *Moves men love*
>
> *"While we were out at dinner, she started playing a little game: She began acting as if we were meeting for the first time on a blind date, asking me questions and flirting with me. At first I thought this was silly, but I played along. Within a few minutes, she lost all of her inhibitions: She told the 'stranger' things she'd never said to me before, and even described what she liked best during sex. I got extremely excited. Playing along with her this way made me feel the thrill of the chase again and got me thinking how badly I wanted to get this 'date' into bed. We had the wildest sex that night—after I begged her to come in to see my CD collection."*
>
> —Neal, 28

helplessness (ditto if he's doing or saying them to you). Once you learn these ropes, maybe you'll feel ready to graduate to some real restraints.

434   Use scarves, neckties, and stockings with caution

They're all handy options, but can tighten during the action and cut off circulation. Plus, the knots in these types of material can be notoriously hard to untie, which is why we highly recommend the following:

435   Keep scissors handy

To snip anything that ends up too tight to untie, of course. Bandage scissors are best, thanks to their blunt lower blade, which will keep you from scraping the skin.

SURPRISING SEX FACT!

On average, women indulge in 14.2 different types of fantasies in a three-month period, according to a study by the *Journal of Sex & Marital Therapy*. Men, though, crave a little more variety, and fantasize an average of 26 different steamy scenarios in the same period of time.

436 Get the right kind of rope

The thicker, the better, as this will make the restraints more comfortable and easier to undo. To avoid rope burns, use cotton rope rather than coarser varieties. Using cuffs? Don't lose the key, cop lady.

437 Tie him up and tease him mercilessly

OK, so you've got him tied spread-eagle on the bed or in a chair with his hands behind his back. What next? Why, it's time to take advantage of his helplessness and tease him into a frenzy. Go down on him until he's about to erupt, then excuse yourself to get a glass of water. Ride him until you're satisfied but leave him hanging until *you* decide he deserves release. The longer you keep satisfaction just out of reach, the better it'll be once you stop torturing the poor guy and let him have it. Talk about a power trip!

Does a little pain hit the spot? Then try these tips...

438   Get a safe word

If you're acting out fantasies that might be painful, scary, or dangerous, a safe word is the seatbelt that will keep your role-play from crashing and burning. Basically, it's a word you both agree upon ahead of time that, if uttered, means things are getting a little *too* crazy for your tastes and that your partner should tone it down or completely call it quits. Make sure to pick a word that you'd never, ever say normally during your scene, like "hippopotamus," "tree," or even plain old "safe word." That way, you can scream, "No!" or "Stop, that hurts!" to your heart's content without one of you worrying, *Um, do they mean it or is it part of the act?*

Girl talk tip-off

"When I finally got up the nerve to ask my guy what his wish was, he said he's always fantasized about me giving him oral sex while he drank single-malt scotch and smoked a cigar. He said it was one of the best nights of his life, and he felt like a king."

—Jamie, 32

439 Set the scene

Stumped on how to segue from your typical Sunday afternoon to a spankfest? Easy: Tell him you caught him spying on you while you were undressing, or you found a porno mag under his bed, or ask him if he's completed some household task on his to-do list you know he hasn't. When he says no, say in a sultry voice he won't mistake, "You've been a very, very bad boy. Come over here so I can teach you a lesson."

440 Keep the pain pleasurable

Steer clear of some obvious no-go zones like the kidneys (the area right above the buttocks) and, of course, the family jewels. If his butt's the bull's-eye, target the fleshy, middle part of each cheek, which can best take a beating. To elicit "Mmm" instead of "Ouch!," start light and watch closely for his reaction. Gently rub the area between each smack, which will increase blood flow and give your spanks a more sensual vibe. Remember, there's a fine line between pleasurable pain and pain pain, so proceed with caution.

SURPRISING SEX FACT!

Out of 40 fantasies mentioned on one survey, both men and women report that (surprise!) intercourse with a loved partner is the most exciting, according to the *Psychological Bulletin*.

Wanna try role-playing? Consider these scenarios...

441 Doctor/patient

Enter his "office" (your bedroom), undress, and tell him: "I have a pain but I'm not sure where it is." Have him examine your body until he finds where it hurts and administers the "cure" (an orgasm). Or he's on his deathbed, and you're in charge of "nursing" him back to health by any means necessary.

442 Boss/employee

You're the head honcho; he's a cute-but-lowly peon. Call him into your office and inform him his "performance" has been lacking of late. He insists he'll do *anything* to keep his job. Now, what do you think that might entail?

443 Stripper/client

Dress in something slinky, don your highest heels, and put on some danceable tunes. Introduce yourself as "Candy" and lead him to a seat, making sure to warn him that club rules are no touching! Then, start gyrating on his lap, shedding layers as you go. (Check out *Carmen Electra's Aerobic Striptease* DVD for inspiration.) Do whatever you can to milk him out of every last dollar in his wallet.

444   Two strangers at a bar

Head separately to a random watering hole—perhaps a place you've never been before to add to the feeling of newness and excitement — and catch his eye at the bar. Let him ply you with Cosmos as he tries to convince you to come back to his place for a nightcap. Make him work for it.

445   Pizza deliveryman/horny housewife

This one's simple: He shows up at your door with a pizza; you invite him in for a slice—and then some.

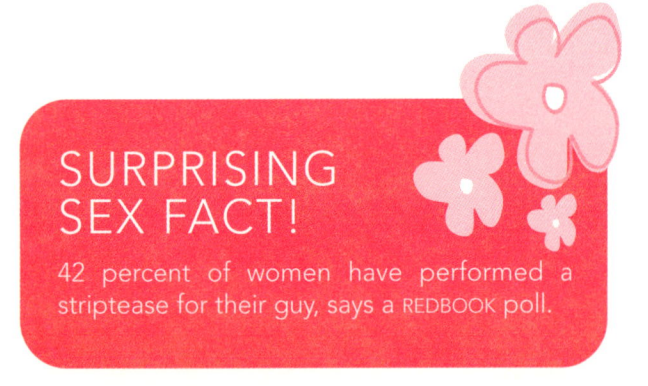

> **SURPRISING SEX FACT!**
>
> 42 percent of women have performed a striptease for their guy, says a REDBOOK poll.

CHAPTER 24

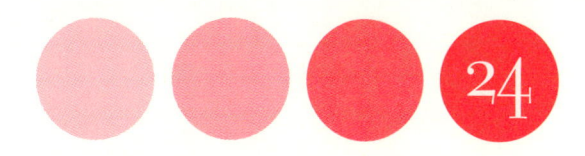

Hey, what about romance?

By this point, you've learned plenty about how to make sex so mind-bogglingly good, you'll need to put on crash helmets before getting busy. But where, you might be wondering, is the romance? Are there specific techniques that can help you hit at the heartstrings and bond emotionally as well as physically? You bet. If you think of sex as a language in which you express how much you love each other, consider this chapter a way to expand your vocabulary and say, "I love you" in all sorts of sensual, soul-moving ways. If it's more intimacy you crave (and who doesn't?), you've come to the right place.

446 Two words: eye contact

This is the simplest trick in the book, and yet much harder than it looks. Given how much your gaze can convey, it's all but impossible to hide anything if you're peeper to peeper. The more you stare, the more you share—so it's bound to bring you closer. If gazing into his baby blues, browns, or hazels feels too intense, try letting your gaze linger on his lips, nose, or forehead and build from there. (Double intimacy points go to those who can manage to maintain eye contact during orgasm.)

447 Write each other forgiveness letters

Let's face it—it's hard to feel lovey-dovey if you're mad at each other, even if it's for tiny, dumb things that have largely blown over. So, it can help to do a little healing before bed by writing each other "forgiveness letters." The letter has to be specific, such as, "When you made that joke about me at Joe and Lisa's party, I felt really embarrassed. I never said anything, but I've been upset with you since then, and I'd like to forgive you." Then he gets to write his own letter. No backtalk or "Yes, but . . . " rejoinders allowed. The point is to say your piece to purge any anger and disappointment you may have been subconsciously hoarding. Do that, and you've cleared the way to a much more intimate evening.

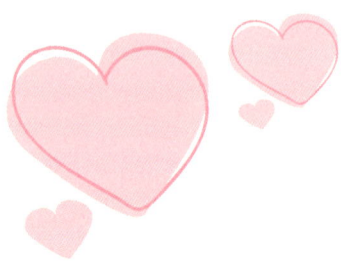

448 During sex, touch him here

No, not *there*. For an intimate rather than erotic effect, caress his face. Run your fingers through his hair. Or, place your hand over his heart to stir some amorous feelings.

449 Make love at half your usual pace

What's the rush? Proceeding in slow-mo will force you to really savor every moment you spend entwined in each other's arms.

450 Tune in to his every breath

Press your cheek to his so his lips are next to your ear, and listen to him inhale and exhale as you make love. Breathing is, after all, as basic as it gets. What better way could there be to get inside his skin and bond on an almost telepathic level?

SURPRISING SEX FACT!

When a REDBOOK poll asked which of three things couples wished they had more of during sex—more foreplay, more experimentation, or more romance—the majority (57 percent) said it's romance they crave.

451 Tell him you want to please him—period . . .

Multitaskers to a fault, many of us tend to give pleasure simultaneously as we're getting it—and feel guilty and self-conscious if we're purely on the receiving end for too long. That's why you should deliberately let your sweetie off the hook one night by saying, "Tonight, I'd like to establish one rule: Let *me* do everything. Don't lift a finger." Ask him what he wants, and allow him to indulge fully in his sensations without being distracted about how you're doing. By showing him he doesn't always have to give to receive, he'll feel truly taken care of. If he resists, tell him, "Don't worry, I'll get you to return the favor soon" (more on that next . . .).

452 . . . Then, switch roles

Next time, tell your guy, "I want you to please me while I kick back"—then let him know where to start. Sounds pretty sweet, but be warned, surrendering in this way can be especially difficult for women, who are often taught to put their own needs last. And when the spotlight's on you, you may feel self-conscious or worry he's getting bored. But the truth is, he's probably at least

---

Moves men love

"Jenna puts her hand over my heart when she reaches orgasm before me. That little move fills me with love—and triggers my own release."

—Jeff, 35

as turned on as you are, since men's egos often hinge on how well they can flip your switch. Allow him to do you this small favor—it's a win-win experience.

> **SURPRISING SEX FACT!**
>
> According to a REDBOOK poll, 76 percent of women say their mates always get some action on their birthday, no matter how tired or stressed they are.

453 Make love with the lights on

No, it's not just about creating some eye candy, but also upping intimacy. In the dark, thoughts drift; your connection can suffer. In the light, your focus will likely remain on what's in front of you: each other.

454 Jump him on a special occasion

Sure, sex for its own sake is always nice. But when it's coupled with a certain pivotal point in life, your romantic moment can resonate on a whole new level (which is why so many couples make a point of getting it on on their anniversary). So pounce on him the day he gets a promotion or, conversely, when he's worn down by a rough week at work. Use sex as a salve or to celebrate, and it'll make the emotional lows not so low and the highs even higher.

455 Pump each other up

Build his self-esteem—and yours—by taking 10 minutes before things heat up to say what you like about each other. Be sure to cover three kinds of compliments: physical ("You have an incredible butt"), appreciative ("I really appreciate that you always pick up the kids"), and emotional ("I feel so safe when I'm in your arms"). Aim for at least one of each, but the more, the merrier. Why? Because the

> **SURPRISING SEX FACT!**
>
> 74 percent of us have ended an argument by tearing each other's clothes off, says a REDBOOK poll.

better you feel about yourselves, the more willing you'll be to share all that you've got to give, in bed and out.

456 Write him a lust note

Similar to a love note but a *lot* racier, this missive will serve as a reminder of five things you adore about him—his strong shoulders, his kissable lips, the sexy way he sighs in bed. The more detailed, the better. Place your note where he can't miss it, like tucked into his coat pocket or behind his shaving cream. Sure, it's sexy, but it's also sweet. After all, when you're showered with compliments, doesn't it make you feel closer to the person who gave them?

457 Never withhold nooky as punishment

For many people—especially women—the phrase "not tonight, honey" is code for *I'm mad at you about something and you're not getting any until we resolve it*. These boycotts, though, are a bad idea. Instead of stewing, speak up if something's still bothering you. By doing so, you keep sex from becoming a bargaining chip in your relationship that will drive you further apart. Instead, it does what it's supposed to: Bring you closer.

458 Better yet, engage in makeup sex

Embroiled in the thick of an argument? We know sex is probably the last thing on your mind right now, but you'd be amazed how quickly your tiff will dissipate if you just reach across that divide, kiss him hard, and take it from there. It conveys in a very powerful, nonverbal way that even though you're miffed, your love isn't on the line. What better way is there to put it all back in perspective?

459 Flash back to a sexy memory

Here's a little-known truth about rabid-for-each-other couples: They're always running a post-game recap of their favorite sexcapades. So, take him to a bar where you first made out and reminisce. Break out your honeymoon album in bed and relive the highlights. By frequently pressing rewind on your most romantic moments, you keep them fresh in your mind—and may trigger more in your future.

One woman's sex secret—revealed

The first time I left the lights on, we were amazed at what we saw. My husband loves looking at my body. But for me it's the intimacy that blows my mind. In the dark it's easy to zone out. We could really focus on each other's expressions, which made the sex so much more personal."

—Annie, 26

460 Try a touch of Tantric sex

No, Tantric sex is *not* a cult ritual that requires you to have sex for eight hours straight. In a nutshell, this ancient practice is a way to forge a spiritual connection. To give it a try, start out by breathing in and out in unison to synchronize your sexual energy. Then, once you've got the hang of that, start alternating inhalations and exhalations—as you breathe in, he breathes out—to create a "circle of breath" that can intensify the arousal. Now, here's the clincher: With regular sex, you let arousal build steadily to a grand finale—but with Tantric sex, you let the sexual energy build *multiple* times by switching back and forth between massage, foreplay, and intercourse, as if these were selections at a buffet rather than a planned-out three-course meal. By the time you're ready to let loose, you should be speaking in tongues—and feeling intensely, spiritually in synch.

Moves men love

"Lola keeps her eyes open during her orgasm. Sometimes she bites her lip, gasps, pants, moans—but she never closes her eyes or turns her head away from me. She gives me everything through her eyes. That is such a gift. And it's so exciting."

—Steve, 36

>> Inside the male mind

"I dig our postromp discussions. No stressy house and work talk, just fun, random stuff. We talk about our kid and what he did that day or if he said anything funny. I get teary-eyed just thinking about it."

—Dan, 31

461 Say his name in bed

After all, his moniker is his most personal possession—and whether it's uttered sweetly or saucily during the throes of passion, it will keep his attention riveted on you rather than drifting off into fantasyland. Maybe it'll encourage him to say *your* name, too, and you'll see what we mean.

462 Make love under the stars

String twinkly Christmas lights around the ceiling of your bedroom, then get hot 'n' heavy under your own private starry sky.

463 Watch him while he's sleeping

This isn't something you can do during sex per se (at least we hope not!), but since you can do it in bed, we figured it's worth mentioning. Try it—there's something about seeing your partner in such a vulnerable state that can foster some warm and fuzzy feelings. And it might just inspire you to give him one heckuva wake-up call.

464 Bring back the pillow talk

Postcoital conversations are a prime time to bond, and when you first started sleeping together you blabbed until dawn. Now, however, these tender moments tend to get extinguished as soon as the sex is over so that you can get some shut-eye or a late-night TV fix. Next time, keep the lights dim and the romance rolling with some ear nibbling, snuggling, and playful conversation. Even if it is just for five minutes, the romantic benefits are immeasurable.

SURPRISING SEX FACT!

22 percent of women say the reason they don't have sex more often is that the guy they're with doesn't want to, according to a REDBOOK poll.

CHAPTER 25

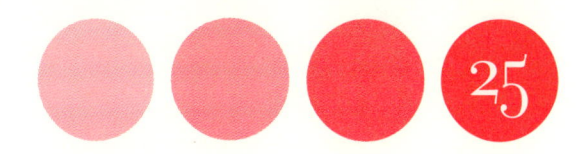

Is your love life MIA?

"Not tonight, honey." Sooner or later, no matter how much we love the guy lying in bed next to us, just about all of us end up uttering those words. How could we not? The daily demands of life—overbearing bosses, whiny kids, a well-meaning partner in crime who can't for the life of him read the directions on a microwavable dinner—aren't exactly mood enhancing. While few admit it openly, many couples' love lives occasionally grind to a halt, where they go weeks, months, or even years without doing the deed. And while one might think women are the ones putting passion on hold, many men, too, would rather zone out to *X-Files* reruns than work up a sweat come bedtime. What gives?

Granted, experts say that a certain ebb and flow is inevitable. But let sex slide for too long and what you've got is (let's be honest here) a roommate rather than a relationship. If you're guilty of hitting the snooze bar on sex one time too many, consider this your wake-up call. Whether you chalk your lagging love life up to a new baby, a busy work schedule, exhaustion, or some mystery cause, we've got answers that'll get romance rolling again and leave your dry spell right where it belongs: in the dust.

Too tired to get it on? Then try these tips...

465 Don't cuddle in bed—instead, embrace standing up

Lying down lulls your body and mind into sleep mode. But you can bypass this response by kissing and canoodling while standing. By the time you two do decide to get horizontal, you'll be too turned on to conk out.

466 Rejigger your carnal clock

Face it: If you keep sex relegated to the dud time slot between the 10 o'clock news and passing out on the pillow, of course your love life's going to suffer. Ditch the restrictive notion that sex is a bedtime ritual, though, and suddenly you'll discover lots of little daily openings to do it in. Try some happy-hour hanky-panky or set the alarm a half hour earlier for one special rise-and-shine that'll keep you floating on air for the rest of the day.

SURPRISING SEX FACT!

According to a REDBOOK survey, 28 percent of women have fallen asleep during sex. (We said we were tired!)

467 Take a few laps up and down the stairs

Getting your blood pumping for even just a few minutes can boost your energy levels and make you more alert. Plus, since increased circulation makes your skin more sensitive, you'll be warming yourself up for a little love before he's even laid a hand on you.

468 Don't exercise too much

Don't get us wrong, *moderate* exercise improves arousal. But if you work out so much you burn more calories than you consume (even if you're trying to lose weight, your body should never run on a calorie deficit), you risk shutting down your pituitary gland, which is responsible not only for keeping your menstrual cycle on track but also for keeping you, well, horny. So make sure you're not overdoing it (30 to 60 minutes several times a week is plenty to reap the arousing benefits).

469 Take turns giving and receiving

Think of all those times you bagged the idea of sex because one of you was too pooped. Now ask yourself this: Who said both partners need to be equally active in bed every time? The next time one of you is raring to go when the other isn't, make a deal that you'll trade off take-charge roles, where the more tired partner just gets to kick back and enjoy the ride. By doing so, you'll double your number of sexcapades without having to exert an ounce more energy than you've got to spare!

Girl talk tip-off

"I used to always succumb to exhaustion when I was home. But now, when I'm tired, instead of shrugging off my husband's seduction attempts, I'll tell myself, Just do it—you'll be glad you did afterward. *And I am. It's taken our lovemaking frequency from once in a while to nearly every day. It's so great to think of sex as a way to connect rather than just another thing on my to-do list."*

—Alix, 33

470 Take the TV out of the bedroom

Admit it: After a long day, it's a lot easier to reach for the remote than for his booty. The TV offers a built-in excuse—er, distraction—lulling you into a passive, nonparticipatory state, which means you're less likely to initiate, engage in, or even *think* about sex. The solution, of course, is simple: Move the TV out of your bedroom. Or at the very least, turn it off and try to come up with some other ways to entertain each other.

471 Spoon your way to sex

If you're *really* too tired to get it on, go ahead and hit the hay—only have him spoon you from behind and (here's the clincher) place his genitals between your legs. Then just fall asleep this way. Feeling your bodies intimately entwined, even while you're slumbering, can have some sexy subliminal effects. Couples who've tried this trick claim they often wake up feeling *very* inspired.

Too stressed for sex? Then try these tips...

472 Write down tomorrow's to-do list before going to bed

Sex requires concentration, and it's no fun to start steaming things up only to entertain thoughts like *Must pick up dry cleaning!* or *Did I spell-check that work memo?* So if there's something looming over you, write it down and vow you'll take care of it tomorrow. That way, you can clear your mind and focus on the present, starting with that hot guy lying next to you.

473 Take time-outs

A mile-long to-do list not only means less time to actually *have* sex, it also floods your body with stress hormones, which dampen your ability to become aroused. The sexy Rx: Take one or two five-minute breaks each day to do something that calms you, whether that's chatting with a friend on the phone or just closing your eyes and taking some deep breaths. A short respite is all it takes to reduce those stress hormones and find your center, sexually and otherwise.

> ### Moves men love
>
> "The alarm clock went off a half hour early one morning, and when I told her it was the wrong time, she smiled, turned it off and said, 'No, it's not.' The rest is history."
>
> —Paul, 38

Girl talk tip-off

"My husband and I have different schedules, so we're not always boiling over with energy at the same times. So we decided that when he's raring to go and I'm utterly beat, he can become the sexual ringmaster for the night. I'll lie back and let him turn me on: There are times when I literally don't raise a finger. It's guilt-free because he knows he'll get the favor returned another night."

—Heather, 39

474 Schedule sex

Sure, you schedule play dates and doctors' appointments and oil changes, but couples are often reluctant to schedule sex because it makes the encounter feel so, well, unsexy. If you worry that having to book an intimate encounter with your man is a sign your romance is dead, consider this: You've been scheduling sex all along. When you were dating, didn't you know you were going to have sex on Saturday night? When you go away to a hotel for a weekend getaway, aren't you certain you're going to be intimate? Bottom line: Penciling in passion doesn't mean you two are boring; it means you're committed to having "just us" time—and what could be more romantic than that?

475 Keep in touch during typically unsexy moments

No one, we repeat, *no one* likes those scarily demonstrative-in-public couples who even feel each other up in the frozen-food aisle. But still, if the only time you're laying your hands on your honey is when you're trying to scoot past him in the kitchen, you're both majorly missing out. There's no harm in hugging for no reason or swapping neck rubs just because. And by physically connecting in small ways throughout the day, you stay warmed up for more intense action later.

476 Assign a sex quota

Every week, agree on the number of times you'll have sex—and promise to meet that goal no matter what. More spontaneous than scheduling date nights, this trick nonetheless guarantees you'll see some action soon enough (or, at the very least, be cramming in a lot of fast and frenzied fun by day seven).

477 Have a shortcut to sex

One of the hardest things to do is transition from, say, paying bills to being sexy with each other. But one easy way to snap each

One woman's sex secret—revealed

"I can't think of a better way to relieve stress than sex. I always think of Annette Bening in American Beauty. *Right after she has sex with Peter Gallagher, she says, 'I really needed that. I was so stressed out!' So true."*

—*Loriann, 30*

other out of daily-grind mode is to develop a secret shorthand for "Let's be sexy together." Maybe your man stretches out on the sofa after the kids are in bed and invites you to hop up next to him. Or you swat his butt, or swap massages. Whatever it is, having a secret sexy code for getting frisky will get things rolling far faster than asking "So how was your day?" and warming up from there.

> **SURPRISING SEX FACT!**
>
> When do couples prefer to get it on? According to a REDBOOK poll, the majority—57 percent—say right before bed; 21 percent prefer sex in the morning; while 16 percent swear nothing beats lazy afternoon lovemaking. And, apparently, 6 percent take "honey, I'm home" to new heights by jumping each other in the evening after work!

478 Consider sex a cure-all

Excuses, excuses—it's so easy to find reasons to put off slipping into the sack. You're busy. You're stressed. You're annoyed and bickering with your husband over something silly. Stop right there and consider what sexy sirens know all too well: that doing the deed can actually *alleviate* stress—the very thing that was supposedly keeping you from getting down in the first place! Once you realize that sex will relax you rather than drain you, you'll find plenty of opportunities to use a little lovin' for an energy boost.

479 Occasionally, make it a quickie

Passionately prolific couples have a philosophy: Frequent sex, no matter what kind, is an absolute must for a good marriage. So if it sometimes has to be a quickie—a.k.a. a fast-and-furious romp without romantic trimmings—so what? It's still good sex. Adopt this attitude, and suddenly your schedule will seem rife with opportunities.

480 Just say no

If you're at the beck and call of your whip-cracking boss or whiny kids, watch out. People who feel like they can't say no to life's demands often try to regain a sense of control where they can—by saying no to sex. If "not tonight, honey" is the only way you're putting your foot down, then maybe it's time instead to start curbing the number of yeses you dole out during your day. Go ahead and say, "Sorry, I can't" to a carpooling buddy who's asking you to swap days on your date night. Or, at the very least, stall by saying, "Hmm, let me check my schedule and get back you." That way, you can avoid a knee-jerk "Sure!" and think about what's best—for you *and* your love life.

Girl talk tip-off

"I write myself notes so I'll remember things, from grocery items to birthdays to checking my stock portfolio. One day after my husband and I had lamented the infrequency of our lovemaking, I wrote 'Sex!' and posted it on the side of my computer monitor. Because that note was there, I thought more about sex than I usually did. I didn't stay late at work that night. We had sex. I left the note up until it fell down. I have replaced the note, and now I've put more notes in my day planner; for example, 'Do it in the pool tonight.'"

—*Donna, 30*

Is a new baby dampening your drive? Here's what to do...

481 See if hormones are to blame

After childbirth, a woman's hormones drop to near post-menopausal levels, which can lower libido. What's more, sometimes they don't recalibrate on their own, especially after a second child. So if your sex drive doesn't bounce back after you give birth, ask your doctor to check your hormone levels (wait six months after you've stopped breastfeeding). If they're low, treatments like testosterone therapy can help.

482 Give your love life a postbaby makeover

Many new moms are reluctant to jump back in the saddle because they're worried sex will feel . . . well . . . different. We won't lie to you: Sometimes it does. Due to the stresses your reproductive organs endured during labor, things may feel looser, or less lubricated, or just plain out of place. You might find that your once tried-and-true

> **SURPRISING SEX FACT!**
>
> How often do couples do it? According to a REDBOOK survey, the majority of us (36 percent) get it on 1 to 2 times per week; 27 percent admit it happens less than once a week. That said, 28 percent manage to squeeze sex in 3 to 5 times a week, while a randy 9 percent make love more than 5 times per week (whew!).

> ## SURPRISING SEX FACT!
> Couples who argue about sex have it more often than those who don't, according to a study by Georgia State University. The reason: Fighting for love shows you care, which breeds warm-and-fuzzy feelings, which then leads to . . . well, we think you know where this is going.

techniques to reach orgasm are no longer flipping your switch. For starters, know that many of these changes to your body are temporary. Until things feel more back to normal, consider this an opportunity to strike out and find *new* moves that'll float your boat. If you're usually a fan of missionary, try hopping on top. Or, if you usually jump straight into intercourse, try oral sex instead. Never tried a vibrator? That might be exactly what your poor sex organs need to rumble back to life. The long and short of it is, your post-baby sexual responses might call for a completely new approach. Seize the opportunity to explore and you may be pleasantly surprised what gets your mojo rising.

483 Clock some girl time

New moms often lose their sense of sexual identity—after all, it's hard to see yourself as a sultry vixen when you've got stretch marks and a baby noshing on your nipples. If you feel like motherhood has eclipsed your formerly fun, free-spirited self, never fear, there *is* a way to reconnect with your womanly side: by hanging out with other women, of course! Call your gal pals for cocktails, coffee, a mani/pedi, or a full-blown day at the spa, and we guarantee you'll come home feeling way more feminine—and that can contribute to your sexual energy.

484 Put a lock on your bedroom door

Once your little munchkins are older, this is a must for your love life. Why? Because without it, your kids could walk in on mommy and daddy in a *very* compromising position at any moment—and this sheer possibility keeps many parents from having sex at all. Why torture yourself? Explain to older kids that you two need some private time and tell them to knock if they need you; if your kids are small, use a monitor so you can get to them quickly. If you think it's cruel to shut the little tykes out, remember: Having a loving sex life is one of the greatest gifts you can give your children, since you're their models for how a healthy intimate life should be—and, with your anxieties about a barge-in banished, you can fully enjoy this parental duty!

>> Inside the male mind

"After my wife had each of our three kids, I encouraged her to go out with the girls. Women need time to reflect with friends; it's given her a clearer view on balancing her emotions about being a lover and mother in the same body. She started coming home much happier and—can I say this?—hornier."

—*Doug, 38*

Is boredom sapping your sex drive? Then try these tips...

485 Exit your comfort zone

Honestly, when's the last time you've tried something new? Go ahead—pop in a porn film, whip out a sex toy, throw a toga party for two. Novelty stimulates the production of dopamine, a brain chemical linked to libido.

486 Return to the basics

For some couples, what's required to spark their libidos isn't novelty at all, but a return to the basics. Kissing. Eye contact. Things a surprising number of couples abandon after they've been together awhile. Try it and you'll see: It sounds simple, but it can get your heart fluttering as if you two had just met.

487 Consider that maybe boredom isn't to blame

Think about it: As your partner becomes more integrated into your life—you buy a home together, combine checking accounts, raise kids—it can become more difficult to take risks sexually since you have more to lose if they reject you. That's why some experts argue that for many couples, boredom isn't what's making sex stale. It's fear. We're not talking quaking-in-your-boots fear, but something much subtler. Ask yourself if you found it easier to be wild 'n' crazy when you didn't know each other as well. If your answer is yes, then you may want to own up to the fact that boredom isn't the whole story here.

What if *he's* not in the mood?
Here's what to do . . .

488 Don't take it personally

Many women take for granted that men are always up for a tumble. But even young guys go through phases when they're lust-challenged: They may be depressed, unhappy with themselves or just plain tired. So, don't make a big deal about it and don't jump to conclusions—chances are, it's *not* because your butt's gotten bigger over the years.

489 Time your talk right

If you want to ask him where his sex drive's disappeared to, *don't* do it right after he's turned you down and you're both feeling vulnerable. Instead, at some other point tell your partner, "I want to talk with you about something Saturday night" or whenever

One woman's sex secret—revealed

"Before giving birth, I'd never been a fan of oral sex (on me) or woman-on-top positions. But I've learned to have a whole new appreciation for them. Childbirth became a springboard to embrace new techniques. It forced us to open up and take chances. And the sex was actually better than when we first dated."

—Holly, 40

> ### Girl talk tip-off
>
> *"Seven years and two kids into our marriage, we became consumed by the chaos of daily responsibilities and let sex slide. We knew it was crucial to find time to be intimate, but the idea of a stock Friday–night–sex date felt too contrived, so we created a variation: Every Monday we pick a random number and have to have sex that many times before the week ends. If three days go by with zero action, we know we've got to make up the time fast. For instance, the other day, while the kids were in the backyard with their grandmother, my husband called me into the garage to help him 'organize a shelf.' But when I got there, he grabbed me and pulled me into the backseat of the car. He said he had no choice since we needed to get busy to make the quota."*
>
> —Eliza, 34

he's free. He may try to jump the gun and get you to tell him now, but wait until you have time for a real heart-to-heart. This is a sensitive topic and shouldn't be rushed.

490 Tackle it as a team

Since questions like "So I've noticed you haven't been jumping me lately—what's wrong with you?" will only put him on the defensive, frame the lack of sex as a problem you're *both* facing. Say, "I noticed *we* haven't been as sexual lately. Is there something you think might be causing this?" Another no-fault con-

> ### Girl talk tip-off
>
> *"We've definitely become that couple who books sex. We work so hard during the week that we're just too exhausted to make love then. So we set aside regular time on Friday and Saturday nights to reconnect and be romantic. We have to make a conscious effort or it just won't happen."*
>
> —Jen, 32

versation tactic is to explain how the lack of intimacy makes you feel, such as lonely or unloved—he can't very well argue with that. Drive home you're unhappy, and your partner should take note and turn a new leaf. If he admits he hasn't been feeling very amorous lately but can't pinpoint the problem, encourage him to get checked out by a doctor. But in most cases, it's normal for him to want to just crash some nights. He's a person, not a porn star!

SURPRISING SEX FACT!

When REDBOOK asked what's keeping women from having sex more often, 14 percent say it's because they are too stressed.

Not sure what the problem is? Then check out these hidden culprits...

491 See if your birth control's to blame

Some birth control pills can drag down libido by increasing—fourfold—the production of a protein that suppresses testosterone, and this effect can last up to a year after you stop taking the Pill, according to a study published in *The Journal of Sexual Medicine*. If you think this is the problem, try forms of contraception that don't contain hormones (like condoms, diaphragms, and certain IUDs).

492 Check the side effects of your antidepressant

Lowered libido is a common side effect among many people who take antidepressants. The biggest culprits: selective serotonin reuptake inhibitors (SSRIs), such as Paxil and Prozac, which boost your body's levels of serotonin, a neurotransmitter that may inhibit your desire for sex. The solution: Switch to one of

> ### Girl talk tip-off
>
> "You have to go with the moment. If the kids are coming home from school in 20 minutes, don't try to light a bunch of candles and dig out your Al Green CD. This is when you nab the window of opportunity and jump on each other. It's done wonders for my sex life and for our marriage."
>
> —Elizabeth, 38

the newer drugs (such as Lexapro or Celexa), or talk to your doctor about taking the antidepressant Wellbutrin in addition to your current medication. Wellbutrin can block your SSRI drug's ability to dampen libido (don't worry, this does not constitute double-dosing on antidepressants; your M.D. can explain).

493 See if he's snoring

If he drones on like a buzz saw all night, that could be a sign he suffers from obstructive sleep apnea, a condition that limits his oxygen intake. Understandably, apnea patients often report they lack the energy or interest for sex. But don't worry, it's usually treatable—and just think, you'll get more sex *and* more sleep!

SURPRISING SEX FACT!

In a perfect world (sans overbearing bosses, crying babies, and other distractions), how often would we ideally like to do it? According to a REDBOOK poll, 45 percent would love a romp every day, with 38 percent wanting it twice as often as the norm, and 17 percent of us content with the amount we have now.

CHAPTER 26

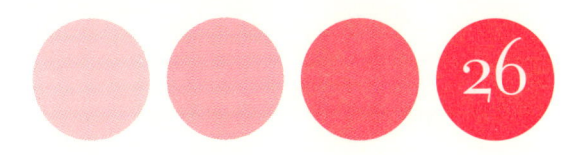

Oops! 7 things you should never, ever try in bed

Now that we've filled your head with hundreds of things you could be doing in bed tonight, we'd feel remiss unless we mentioned a few things we recommend couples *don't* try anytime soon. As for why, look no further than these cautionary tales from women who actually committed these slip-ups and were willing to spill the details. Let their stories serve as reminders that no matter how accomplished you are between the sheets, sex is full of surprises—sometimes painful, embarrassing ones—but provided no one suffers any permanent injuries, you have to admit it's pretty funny. So please, go ahead and have a laugh at these ladies' expense, learn from their mistakes, and remember that no couple should be taking sex *too* seriously. If we can't throw in a few giggles along with those sighs, moans, and ohmigods, sex wouldn't be half as much fun.

494 Don't record this on your outgoing message

"One time while my husband and I were making love, my cat walked on top of our answering machine. Little did we know that she had stepped on some buttons and rerecorded our outgoing message. It was almost a week before we realized that anyone who called us and got the machine was being treated to the glorious sounds of love."

—Amy, 29

495 Don't leap before you look

"We had been married only two months when my husband decided to take a running leap onto our bed, where I was sitting seductively. Imagine my surprise when he landed on my knee and I heard something snap! A trip to the doctor confirmed that I had torn a ligament, and I ended up in a wheelchair for the next month. Our friends teased us mercilessly because they knew that when we first started dating, my oh-so-graceful husband had also dislocated my middle finger with one of his flying leaps."

—Pippa, 28

496 Don't heat things up too much

"Hoping to surprise my honey, I packed the kids off to their grandparents' and set up a romantic picnic in our living room. I thought caramel would be sexy to eat (and play with), so I heated some up in our fondue pot. As we lay on a picnic blanket by candlelight, I grabbed a slice of apple, dipped it into the sweet stuff, and allowed some of the sauce to drizzle on him, which I was planning to kiss off. But before I even had a chance to get a taste, my hubby started screeching because the sizzling sauce was burning his chest. He hasn't let me bring any (hot) food near him ever since."

—Lisa, 36

497 Don't go wild when the walls are thin

"I went with my man and his family to a New Year's party at a beach resort. After a few too many drinks, we went back to our room and had a very passionate (and noisy) night. The next morning I was a little hung over, so my boyfriend went across the hall to his aunt and uncle's room for some aspirin. That's when I noticed I could hear every word he was saying. Then it got worse: Coming from across the hall were the sounds of his relatives laughing as his aunt mimicked me screaming out my boyfriend's name. Talk about humiliation—and thin walls!"

—Kelly, 31

498 Don't be rash

"To spice up our routine, I bought some flavored massage oil for my husband and me to try. We put an old sheet down in the living room and started to massage each other with the oil. So far so good! But a few minutes into our session, we both started itching like crazy because of some allergic reaction to the oil. All that scratching made us so miserable that we had to hit the shower—effectively cooling off what had started out as a sexy encounter."

—Kristin, 35

499 Don't snort this

"I bought a new bottle of body lotion with the intention of giving my sweetie a sensual massage. To get a whiff of the yummy scent, I squeezed the bottle and ended up squirting a glob of lotion right up my nose! My husband's hysterical laughter kind of put a damper on the mood."

—Dawn, 33

500 Don't fall completely head over heels

"One night I decided to do a striptease for my boyfriend. I put on my sexiest teddy and stood up on the end of the bed to give him a better view. Everything was going great until I tried to slip off the teddy. I slid it down to my ankles, but as I tried to seductively kick it off, I lost my balance and rolled backward off the bed, landing flat on my tush. I knew he was marriage material when he checked to make sure I was all right before giggling at my super-suave move. Now, 12 happily married years later, just thinking about that incident still cracks us up."

—Michele, 32

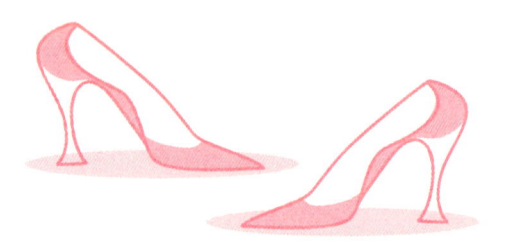

Sources

For sex toys:
goodvibes.com
babeland.com

For female-friendly porn:
candidaroyalle.com

For sex therapy:
aasect.org
passionatemarriage.com

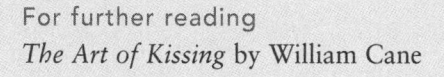

For further reading

The Art of Kissing by William Cane

The Big O: Orgasms: How to Have Them, Give Them, and Keep Them Coming by Lou Paget

The Essence of Tantric Sexuality by Mark Michaels and Patricia Johnson

For Women Only, Revised Edition: A Revolutionary Guide to Reclaiming Your Sex Life by Jennifer Berman, Laura Berman, and Elisabeth Bumiller

He Comes Next: The Thinking Woman's Guide to Pleasuring a Man by Ian Kerner, Ph.D.

How to Be a Dominant Diva by Georgia Payne and Julie Taylor

How to Be a Great Lover: Girlfriend-to-Girlfriend Totally Explicit Techniques that Will Blow His Mind by Lou Paget

How to Give Her Absolute Pleasure: Totally Explicit Techniques Every Woman Wants Her Man to Know by Lou Paget

How to Tell a Naked Man What to Do by Candida Royalle

The Passion Prescription: Ten Weeks to Your Best Sex—Ever! by Laura Berman

Rekindling Desire: A Step-by-Step Program to Help Low-Sex and No-Sex Marriages by Barry W. McCarthy and Emily J. McCarthy

The Secrets of Happily Married Men: Eight Ways to Win Your Wife's Heart Forever by Scott Haltzman and Theresa Foy

Secrets of the Sexually Satisfied Woman: Ten Keys to Unlocking Ultimate Pleasure by Laura Berman, Jennifer Berman, and Alice Burdick Schweiger

She Comes First: The Thinking Man's Guide to Pleasuring a Woman by Ian Kerner, Ph.D.

Index

Alcohol and drinking, 65, 80, 81, 192
Anal stimulation and sex, 120, 126, 130, 134, 171, 211
Baby, new, 240–242
Beach sex, 192
Benefits of sex, 10–11
Bondage, 214–216
Boredom, 243
Bras. *See* Lingerie and undies
Brazilian wax, 50
Breasts, 33, 35, 76, 156, 177, 195, 203. *See also* Cleavage; Nipples
Car, sex in/on, 197–198
Cleavage, 34, 37, 47, 210
Clitoral area, 122, 129–133, 146–150, 152, 153, 154, 156, 157, 165, 167, 171, 186, 187, 189
Clothing, 43–52, 75, 84, 87, 89, 102–103, 198. *See also* Striptease and nudity
Communicating about sex, 16, 201–206. *See also* Fantasies
romance and, 221–230
Dancing, 56, 70, 77, 78, 132, 209. *See also* Striptease and nudity
Dates, 67–82
   ideas for going out, 68–75
   ideas for staying in, 75–82
Decorating tips, 39–42
Erogenous zones, 107–116. *See also* Hot spots
Exercise (sexercise), 53–59, 233
Fantasies, 207–220
   bondage, 214–216
   making come true, 213–214
   pain, 217–218
   role-playing, 219–220
   talking about, 208–213
Flirting, 25, 30, 36, 90, 215
Foods and eating, 60–66, 68–69, 74
Foreplay, 101–106
G-spot, 130, 132–133, 163, 171
G-spot, male, 120, 125
Hair, 45, 46, 50
Hammock, sex on, 199–200
Hand jobs (for her), 127–134
Hand jobs (for him), 117–126
Hints, dropping, 82, 87, 92, 195–196
Hot spots. *See also* Erogenous zones
   hers, 129–130, 144, 146, 166, 171
   his, 105–106, 120, 122, 166
Humorous things to avoid, 249–252
Intercourse
   orgasms and, 161–174
   places to have. *See* Locations for sex
   positions, 151–160
   romance and, 221–230
   sexy surprises, 175–184
Jacuzzi, sex in, 194–195
Kegels, 57–58
Kissing, 35, 37, 88, 93–100, 103, 106, 110, 113, 114, 157, 177, 212, 227, 232, 243
Lack of sex solutions, 231–248
   boredom and, 243
   fatigue and, 232–234
   getting her in mood, 19–30
   getting him in mood, 19–38, 244–246
   myth about, 17–18
   new baby and, 240–242
   stress and, 235–239
   troubleshooting

index

problems, 247–248
Lingerie and undies, 35, 38, 44, 45, 46, 47, 49, 51, 74, 81, 85, 86, 88, 172, 197
Locations for sex, 191–200
  beach, 192
  car, 197–198
  hammock, 199–200
  Jacuzzi, 194–195
  office, 200
  outdoors, 197
  plane, 193
  shower, 195–196
  waterbed, 198–199
Lubrication, 65, 118–119, 124, 126, 128, 134, 194, 196
Making up and make-up sex, 222, 227
Massage, 27–28, 102, 103, 111–112, 123, 228, 238, 251–252
Masturbating, 121, 128–129, 163, 164, 166, 203, 208
Mood
  getting her in, 19–30
  getting him in, 19–38, 244–246
  making it happen, 12. *See also* Lack of sex solutions
Moves to make, 83–92
Movies, 26, 37, 49, 71, 73, 77, 79, 92, 182, 211
Music, 40, 56, 76, 78, 219
Myths, 9–18
Never dos, 249–252
Nipples, 105, 112, 241
N-spot, 110
Office, sex at, 200
Oral sex
  for (to) her, 143–150, 171
  for (to) him, 135–142
Orgasms, 161–174
Outdoor sex, 197
Pain, as fantasy, 217–218
Peeks, surprise and sneak, 33, 37, 38, 74
Plane, sex on, 193
Positions, 151–160
  challenging, 158–160
  from behind, 155
  her on top, 154
  missionary variations, 152–153
  sideways, 156–157
Pubic hair, trimming or waxing, 50, 137, 144
Role-playing, 219–220
Romance, 221–230
Scheduling sex, 236
Sensory stimulation, 29
Sex drive problems. *See* Lack of sex solutions
Sex toys, 185–190. *See also* Vibrators
Sex, what it is, 15
Showering and bathing, 24, 32, 42, 78, 79, 80, 84, 87, 89, 103, 118–119, 192, 195–197
Smoking, 128, 137, 216
Sources, 253–254
Stress, 235–239
Striptease and nudity, 27, 33, 38, 46, 63, 81, 86, 102–103, 219, 252
Surprises, sexy, 175–184
Tantric sex, 228
Testicles, 125, 141–142
Time for sex, 13–14. *See also* Lack of sex solutions
Touching and caressing, 38, 44, 72, 102–105, 117–126, 127–134, 148, 171, 179, 206, 223, 237. *See also* Erogenous zones; Hot spots
Toys, 185–190. *See also* Vibrators
Trigasm, 171
Vaginal area, 27, 57, 118, 129, 130, 131, 132–134, 149, 152, 155, 163, 178, 186, 189. *See also* Clitoral area; G-spot
Vibrators, 163, 173, 185, 186–187, 188, 189, 190, 241
Waterbed, 198–199
Whispering, 32, 37, 169, 202, 204